COMBINED IMMUNODEFICIENCY DISEASE AND ADENOSINE DEAMINASE DEFICIENCY

A Molecular Defect

BIRTH DEFECTS INSTITUTE SYMPOSIA

Ernest B. Hook, Dwight T. Janerich, and Ian H. Porter, editors:
MONITORING, BIRTH DEFECTS AND ENVIRONMENT:
The Problem of Surveillance, 1971

Ian H. Porter and Richard G. Skalko, editors: HEREDITY AND
SOCIETY, 1972

Dwight T. Janerich, Richard G. Skalko, and Ian H. Porter, editors:
CONGENITAL DEFECTS: New Directions in Research, 1973

*Hilaire J. Meuwissen, Richard J. Pickering, Bernard Pollara, and
Ian H. Porter, editors:* COMBINED IMMUNODEFICIENCY
DISEASE AND ADENOSINE DEAMINASE DEFICIENCY: A
Molecular Defect, 1975

In preparation
S. Kelly, E. B. Hook, D. T. Janerich, and I. H. Porter, editors:
BIRTH DEFECTS: RISKS AND CONSEQUENCES

ACADEMIC PRESS RAPID MANUSCRIPT REPRODUCTION

COMBINED IMMUNODEFICIENCY DISEASE AND ADENOSINE DEAMINASE DEFICIENCY

A Molecular Defect

Edited by

Hilaire J. Meuwissen
Birth Defects Institute
New York State Department of Health
Albany, New York

Bernard Pollara
Birth Defects Institute
New York State Department of Health
Albany, New York

Richard J. Pickering
Children's Hospital
Dalhousie University
Halifax, Nova Scotia
Canada

Ian H. Porter
Birth Defects Institute
New York State Department of Health
Albany, New York

Associate Editors

Ernest B. Hook
Birth Defects Institute
New York State Department of Health
Albany, New York

Sally Kelly
Birth Defects Institute
New York State Department of Health
Albany, New York

Proceedings of a Symposium and Workshop on
Combined Immunodeficiency Disease and Adenosine Deaminase Deficiency:
A Molecular Defect
Sponsored by the Birth Defects Institute of the
New York State Department of Health
Held in Albany, New York, October 2-3, 1973

Academic Press, Inc.
New York   San Francisco   London
A Subsidiary of Harcourt Brace Jovanovich, Publishers

1975

ACADEMIC PRESS, INC.
111 Fifth Avenue, New York, New York 10003

United Kingdom Edition published by
ACADEMIC PRESS, INC. (LONDON) LTD.
24/28 Oval Road, London NW1

Library of Congress Cataloging in Publication Data
Main entry under title:

Combined immunodeficiency disease and adenosine deami-
    nase deficiency, a molecular defect.

    (Birth Defects Institute symposia)
    Bibliography: p.
    Includes index.
        1.   Immunological deficiency syndromes–Congresses.
2.   Adenosine deaminase–Congresses.   I.   Meuwissen,
Hilaire J., ed.   II.   Birth Defects Institute.
III.   Series: Birth Defects Institute.   Symposia.
[DNLM: 1.   Adenosine–Metzbolism–Congresses.
2.   Deficiency diseases–Congresses.   3.   Immunologic
deficiency syndromes–Congresses.   QW504 C631 1973]
RC578.C65   616.07'9   75-4603
ISBN 0–12–492750–5

PRINTED IN THE UNITED STATES OF AMERICA

CONTENTS

CONTENTS

SECTION III

SECTION IV

CONTENTS

SECTION V

CONTENTS

PARTICIPANTS

Arthur J. Ammann, University of California, San Francisco, California

Flossie Cohen, Children's Hospital of Michigan, Detroit, Michigan

Irving H. Fox, Wellesley Hospital, Toronto, Canada

Park S. Gerald, Children's Hospital, Boston, Massachusetts

Eloise R. Giblett, King County Central Blood Bank, Seattle, Washington

A. J. Glasky, New Port Pharmaceutical Company, Newport Beach, California

Howard Green, Massachusetts Institute of Technology, Cambridge, Massachusetts

John W. Hadden, Sloan-Kettering Institute, New York, New York

Kurt Hirschhorn, Mt. Sinai School of Medicine, New York City, New York

Rochelle Hirschhorn, New York University Medical Center, New York, New York

Richard Hong, University of Wisconsin, Madison, Wisconsin

R. G. Keightley, University Hospital, Birmingham, Alabama

Stephen D. Litwin, The New York Hospital-Cornell Medical Center, New York, New York

PARTICIPANTS

Hilaire J. Meuwissen, Birth Defects Institute, New York State Department of Health, Albany, New York

Ellen C. Moore, Birth Defects Institute, New York State Department of Health, Albany, New York

William L. Nyhan, University of California, San Diego, California

Richard J. Pickering, Children's Hospital, Dalhousie University, Halifax, Nova Scotia, Canada

Bernard Pollara, Kidney Disease Institute, New York State Department of Health, Albany, New York

Ian H. Porter, Director, Birth Defects Institute, New York State Department of Health, Albany, New York

Newton Ressler, University of Illinois Medical Center, Chicago, Illinois

Fred S. Rosen, Children's Hospital, Boston, Massachusetts

Diane W. Wara, University of California, San Francisco, California

Justin J. Wolfson, University of Wisconsin, Madison, Wisconsin

PREFACE

In 1972, two children with combined immunodeficiency disease were described who lacked detectable adenosine deaminase activity in their red cells. The association between these two rare entities was thought to be significant and led to the organization of a Workshop as part of the annual Birth Defects Symposium which was held in Albany, New York, in October 1974. The proceedings of these meetings form the contents of this book.

Data on more than 80 patients were submitted for evaluation at the Workshop by physicians from all over the world; 12 patients with combined immunodeficiency disease were found to have adenosine deaminase deficiency in their red cells. The data from these patients, and from a group of children with combined immunodeficiency disease and normal adenosine deaminase activity in their red cells, form the basis of this study. Participants in the Workshop concluded that patients with adenosine deaminase deficiency and combined immunodeficiency disease have a syndrome with characteristic clinical, radiologic, and histologic features. Also the data clarified the genetic control of adenosine deaminase, established the pattern of inheritance of adenosine deaminase deficiency, and provided convincing evidence for a causal relationship between the enzyme deficit and the immunologic disorder. The fruitful outcome of the Workshop was due in large part to the collaboration between clinicians, immunologists, geneticists and biochemists at these meetings.

Many people contributed to the success of the Workshop and the Symposium. In particular, we would like to thank Mr. Edwin C. Jones, Mrs. Rosemary Null, Mrs. Ellen J. Heenehan, and many other members of the New York State Health Department Birth Defects and Kidney Disease Institutes for their spontaneous, generous and expert help.

SECTION I

GENES AND DISEASE

Ian H. Porter

Introduction

We have met to discuss the significance of the discovery of the first primary immunodeficiency disorder with an enzyme defect. This will almost certainly be followed by the discovery of (1) more examples of immunodeficiency disorders as inborn errors of metabolism and (2) considerable heterogeneity within this group of disorders. By way of introduction, therefore, I would like to explain the principles which underly the seemingly endless diversity of human traits and conditions.

Ideally, we should be able to relate any inherited condition to a specific gene. Indeed, a full account of any given characteristic should start by determining the sequence of those amino acids in the enzyme that the gene controls, proceed to elucidate the effect of the enzyme on the appropriate biochemical pathway and then correlate this with the clinical picture.

Often, of course, we do this in the reverse order by making clinical observations and then subjecting the questions put to us by these "experiments of nature" to analysis in the laboratory. It is by this method that genetics has made such an important impact on the clinical sciences on the one hand and the basic sciences on the other.

Mutation

DNA has two characteristics: it is remarkably stable and it replicates identically. If this were not true, the orderly development of an individual and the stability of a species would not be possible. If, on the other hand, we were all identical, then the question of inheritance might never have arisen because it is the differences which provide us with the observational units in genetics. One of the causes of individual variation is mutation which leads to a change in one code word. Once a gene has changed it is, of course, preserved in its new state. A gene is made up of code words which consist of trios of DNA nucleotides each of which specifies a given amino acid in that sequence of amino acids which makes up an enzyme. So, if an enzyme is made up of 100 amino acids, then that gene which specifies this enzyme must be

3

made up of 300 nucleotides, each of which is potentially equally mutable. A mutation of any one of these nucleotides will result in one of the amino acids of the enzyme being substituted for another. As a result, the enzyme will be altered. Some of these changes may not have much effect on enzyme activity, some may lead only to slight variation, while others may cause disease or even be lethal. So we can, in a way, say that human genetics is the study of individual variation and medical genetics is a study of those differences which lead to disease. In other words, the differences in the genotype, which under certain conditions lead to disease, are merely a selective sample of all the differences that make each one of us unique.

It is not yet possible to define the abnormality in any genetic condition by direct examination of the sequence of the DNA bases in the gene involved. But we can deduce the change in DNA by isolating the abnormal protein or enzyme and determining the structural defect. For example, in sickle cell disease, the various clinical and pathological features are due to the synthesis of an abnormal hemoglobin which differs from the normal only in one single amino acid; i.e., at the 6th position of the β polypeptide chain at which point valine replaces glutamic acid. Almost all the findings in sickle cell disease can be explained by the physical properties of reduced hemoglobin S, particularly by its low small region on the surface of the protein molecule by the substitution of the hydrophobic valine for the hydrophilic glutamic residue. As the normal β chain is made up of 146 amino acids and as each amino acid is coded for by a trio of bases, the gene determining that chain must contain 438 bases, there could, theoretically, be 438 hemoglobin variants in the β chain alone, some of which would have little in the way of clinical effects and some which would produce serious disease (Fig. 1).

Now, when we talk about genes, there appear to be two kinds: structural ones, which determine the structure of the polypeptides and regulator ones, which determine their rate of synthesis. Based on bacterial systems, we might envisage the operon as the unit which controls and coordinates the synthesis of functionally related proteins. The operator gene is usually closely situated to a group of structural genes, whereas the regulator gene may be some distance removed from this unit. Despite voluminous discussion of structural versus regulatory gene mutations in man, as yet no well-documented examples of the latter are comparable to the operon in bacterial systems. For example, the decreased rate of synthesis in β chains of hemoglobins in thalassemia has been proposed as an example of a regulator gene defect but it is much more likely to reside in the rate of translation of the mRNA. Acute intermittent porphyria was another candidate for regulatory mutation because of the increased activity of δ-aminolevulinic acid (ALA) synthetase but this can probably also be explained on the basis of structural gene mutation by analogy with the

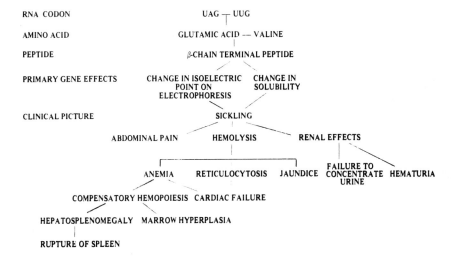

Fig. 1. Pedigree of causes for sickle cell disease.

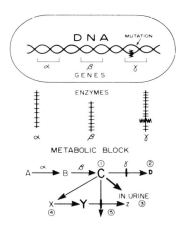

Fig. 2. Diagrammatic representation of an inborn error of metabolism.

Hektoen variant of glucose-6-phosphate dehydrogenase (G6PD) which is associated with an increase in enzyme activity and in which a structural gene mutation has been demonstrated. In other words, we cannot yet predict the effect that an amino acid substitution will have on enzyme behavior.

Inborn Errors of Metabolism

A mutation then is a simple base substitution in DNA leading to a single amino acid substitution in an enzyme. This may so alter the properties of the enzyme involved that the enzyme responsible for a metabolic step may be blocked with the following consequences (Fig. 2):

1. high levels in the serum of the substrate proximal to the metabolic block,
2. a deficiency in the serum of the product distal to the block,
3. excess excretion in the urine of the substrate, and
4. secondary metabolic block.

Thus, in phenylketonuria (PKU), the absence of phenylalanine hydroxylase activity leads to an accumulation of phenylalanine in the serum, a block in tyrosine formation and an increased urinary excretion of phenylpyruvic and other acids. The high concentrations of phenylalanine causes a suppression of tyrosine activity which leads to a defect in melanin formation resulting in decreased pigmentation. Thus, an inborn error of metabolism is a disease in which characteristic clinical, pathological and biochemical abnormalities can be attributed to the congenital alteration of the activity of a specific enzyme, which in turn is due to the presence of a particular abnormal gene. The corollary of this is, of course, that genes control all metabolic processes.

As genes control metabolic pathways and as mutations occur constantly and randomly — that is to say, all parts of the genetic material are equally susceptible — we might in time expect to discover an increasing number of inborn errors of metabolism. Thus, for example, in the pathway for the degradation of phenylalanine and tyrosine we know of four metabolic blocks involving sequential steps in that metabolic pathway — phenylketonuria, tyrosinosis, alkaptonuria and albinism; in the Embden-Meyerhof pathway we know of ten metabolic blocks produced by enzyme deficiencies involving sequential steps in the pathway of red cell glucose metabolism; and in the metabolic pathway involved in cortisol production we know of seven different metabolic blocks leading to various forms of the congenital adrenal hyperplasia syndromes.[1] At the present time, there are about 110 known inborn errors of metabolism in which the enzyme has been identified and the rate of discovery of inborn errors of metabolism is increasing. There could, indeed, be a variation — if not a disease — associated with every enzyme responsible for every step in every metabolic pathway. It is estimated that if the present rate of discovery continues there will be about 12,000 known inborn errors of metabolism in the year 2009 – the centenary of the publication of Sir Archibald Garrod's *Inborn Errors of Metabolism* (Fig. 3).[2]

Allelism

Mutations may not only involve genes at different loci controlling different metabolic steps in the same or different metabolic pathways, but also different bases within the same gene and the randomness of mutations predicts that not only may all genes be affected but so, also, may each nucleotide in each gene. Thus, a large number of different mutual alleles may be generated from a single gene by separate mutational events. For example, from a gene containing a sequence of DNA 900 bases long and coding for an enzyme of 300 amino acids, 2,700 different alleles each differing from the original by only a single base change may be formed by separate mutations, since each of the 900 bases may be altered to one of three others in different mutational events. Some 20-25%, however, of all mutations of this type will be synonymous. That is to say, they will result in no alteration in the amino acid structure of the enzyme because they will simply involve the change of a particular codon to another specifying the same amino acid. In about four percent of cases, mutation will cause an alteration of a base triplet coding for an amino acid to a nonsence triplet which results in chain termination. The mutant allele will then cause the synthesis of a shortened polypeptide chain lacking a greater or lesser proportion of its carboxyl terminal amino acid sequence. This is likely to result in considerable disruption of protein structure with loss of functional activity.

In some 70-75% of cases, a single base change will result in the synthesis of an enzyme differing from the original by the substitution of one amino acid for another at the corresponding point in its amino acid sequence. Since each of the several hundred amino acids in an enzyme may be changed to one of several others by such mutations, a considerable variety of structurally different variants may be produced in this way and we find that there is a wide range of diversity of phenotypes which can be produced by allelic series. Genes known to be allelic because they determine structural variants of the β chain of hemoglobin produce phenotypes as disparate as cyanosis in Hemoglobin M$_{Saskatoon}$, polycythemia in Hemoglobin Malmö, persistent anemia in Hemoglobin S or intermittent anemia precipitated by drugs in Hemoglobin Zürich. If it were not for biochemical evidence of allelism, these conditions would probably be considered determined by genes at different loci. Further diversity is provided when two different rare alleles are present at the same locus: for example, hemoglobin SC is distinct from both homozygous SS and CC. In compound heterozygotes (the presence of two different alleles at the *same* locus as opposed to a double heterozygote

7

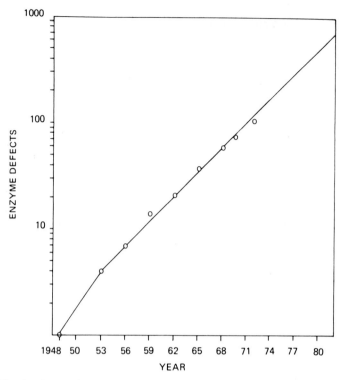

Fig. 3. Rate of increase for the discoveries of inborn errors of metabolism (by permission of the author and publisher).[3]

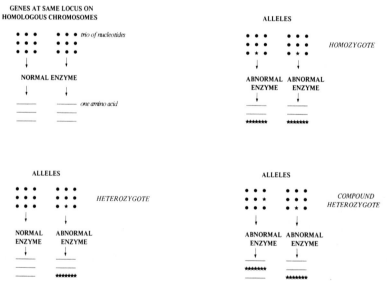

Fig. 4. Diagrammatic representation of allelism.

which is the presence of two different alleles at *different* loci) an increased frequency of parental consanguinity is neither expected nor seen (Fig. 4). As another example there are about 80 known different variants of glucose-6-phosphate dehydrogenase and they can be attributed to different mutant alleles at a single locus on the X-chromosome and they also are different from one another in their clinical consequences. Some give rise to persistent hemolytic disease and are analogous to the enzyme variants found in inborn errors of metabolism, others produce no clinical abnormality under ordinary conditions but render the individual particularly susceptible to certain drugs, and still others appear to have no adverse effects at all. It turns out that if we investigate any enzyme there are usually one or two common variants in the population (frequencies greater than 1:1,000) and then there are usually a number of rare ones (frequencies less than 1:10,000). These findings imply that any single individual may be heterozygous at about 16% of all gene loci coding for the structures of enzymes. If there are 50,000 structural genes — which is perhaps a conservative estimate — one would expect that in any single person there may be about 8,000 loci at which there are two different alleles resulting in the synthesis of a structurally distinct form of a particular enzyme or protein.[4]

Modes of Inheritance

Most of the inborn errors of metabolism are inherited as autosomal or X-linked recessive conditions (Fig. 5, 6). Affected individuals with typical clinical and metabolic features of the disease are homozygotes (or hemizygotes in the case of males in the X-linked conditions) for the particular gene while their parents or their mother, as the case may be, are heterozygotes (carriers). There is often consanguinity in these families and the rarer the incidence of the disease, the higher the incidence of consanguinity. In view of the extraordinary degree of genetic variation, it now looks as if true homozygotes for rare conditions may *only* arise from consanguineous marriages and that those apparent homozygotes resulting from the beds of unrelated marriages are more likely to be the result of compound heterozygotes from different alleles.

Although carriers are quite healthy, they usually have partial enzyme deficiency and exhibit minor metabolic disturbances which, for example, can be brought out by stress tests, of which the phenylalanine loading test is a well known example.

In view of the small family size, it is quite common for only one member of a sibship to be involved and although these are sometimes referred to as sporadic cases it does not, of course, imply that they are not hereditary. For example, if you take 16 two child families, in whom the parents are known to

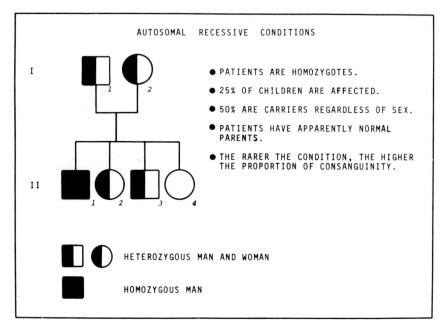

Fig. 5. Characteristics of recessive conditions.

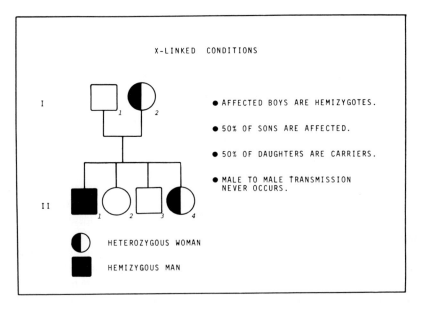

Fig. 6. Characteristics of X-linked conditions.

be carriers, only 7 will be ascertained because they have affected children. In other words, there are a large number of couples in the population who are at risk for having affected children who do not, in fact, have them.

Summary

This is the first time that an immune disorder has been shown to be associated with an inborn error of metabolism and we can now begin to draw a so-called pedigree of causes analogous to the one for hemoglobin S (Fig. 7). During the next few years we will almost certainly find variants of ADA analogous to hemoglobin and G6PD and, in addition, we will almost certainly find heterogeneity of the combined immunological deficiency (CID) syndromes based on involvement of different genes responsible for the production of different enzymes controlling different steps in the purine or other metabolic pathways.[5] Heterogeneity of the CID syndromes has, of course, already been established in that those patients with ADA deficiency look as if they have an autosomal recessive condition and that, at least, some of those patients with CID syndrome with normal ADA activity have an X-linked condition. They must, in other words, be determined by different genes. Further, my guess would be that only the few ADA deficient patients who are the result of consanguineous marriages are truly homozygous and that the rest are compound heterozygotes representing an array of different alleles.

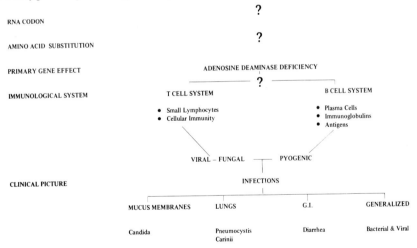

Fig. 7. Pedigree of causes for ADA deficiency in combined immunologic deficiency disease.

REFERENCES

1. M.I. New and L.S. Levine, *Advances Hum. Genet. 4,* 251, 1973.

2. B. Childs, *in* Genetics and the Perinatal Patient, Mead Johnson Symposium on Perinatal and Developmental Medicine, No. 1, p. 39, 1972.

3. V.A. McKusick, *Amer. J. Hum. Genet. 25,* 446, 1973.

4. H. Harris, *in* Human Genetics Excerpta Medica, J. de Grouchy, F.J.G. Ebling and I.W. Henderson (Eds.), p. 273, Amsterdam, 1972.

5. J.B. Stanbury, J.B. Wyngaarden and D.S. Fredrickson, The Metabolic Basis of Inherited Disease, 3rd Edition, McGraw-Hill Book Co., pp. 1778, 1972.

6. V.A. McKusick, Mendelian Inheritance in Man, 3rd Edition, The Johns Hopkins Press, Baltimore and London, pp. 738, 1971.

7. M. Lesch, *N. Engl. J. Med. 283,* 1221, 1970.

GENETIC CONTROL OF GAMMAGLOBULINS*

Stephen D. Litwin

To understand the levels of genetic control imposed on human immuno-globulin (Ig), it is necessary to examine: i) the type of genes involved in Ig synthesis and immune response; ii) the biologic features of these genes; iii) the interrelationship of the above to defects in the immune system of man. This discussion will consider (I) *structural*, (II) *immune response* and (III) *control* genes. The term "control gene" is not applied in a strict sense and refers to genetically determined control of the immune response not clearly associated with Ig structural genes or histocompatibility linked immune response (Ir) loci.[1]

I. *Structural genes* determine the amino acid constitution and sequence of a protein. Genetically determined antigens on human γ (Gm) and a (Am) heavy chains and k light chains (Inv) serve as markers for Ig structural genes in man. These antigens are detected by inhibition of a hemagglutination reaction. The critical antibodies for genetic typing, capable of recognizing Gm antigens, are found in the blood of patients with rheumatoid arthritis and in rare normal sera, or are elicited by animal immunization.[2]

The Gm markers for γ heavy chains in man have proven most informative[2] and will be discussed in further detail.

Gm markers have been *localized* by immunochemical methods to amino acids at various positions in the constant region of the γ chain. In one instance, multiple genetic antigens, Gm(a) an Fc marker and Gm(z) an Fd marker, have been found on the same IgG1 heavy chains (in Caucasians) and appear to be controlled by a single or by linked genes.[3] In rabbits, allotypic markers located in the constant and variable regions of the heavy chain segregate as a single genetic unit.[4] Gm markers can be specified by as little as a

*This work was aided by grants from the United States Public Health Service (A1-09239 and AM-202122).

single amino acid. Examples of this are Gm(f) located at amino acid 214 and Gm(a) at the amino acids 356 or 358. In addition to the primary structure of the Gm antigen, the expression of Gm factors is influenced by the tertiary configuration of the intact IgG molecule. As a rule, Fd antigens cannot be detected on the isolated heavy chain subunit whereas Fc Gm factors are relatively unaffected.[2]

Analysis of the *genetic transmission* of Gm characters in families has demonstrated that they are co-dominant traits, determined by genes on autosomal chromosomes. When Gm markers were used in conjunction with Inv markers of k light chains, it was found that γ heavy chains and k light chains were not linked. In addition, animal studies indicate that λ chains are a third *independent* linkage group of Ig allotype genes. To date, attempts to show a relationship between any of the above structural Ig genes and other known genetic markers have proven fruitless with the exception of a linkage between a-1-antitrypsin and Gm systems.[5]

To understand the formal genetics of the more than 20 Gm factors already described, it is necessary to correlate the genetic antigens with the four subclasses of γ heavy chains present in all normal sera (Table 1). Subclasses differ from each other in a limited portion of their primary structure as well as in biological properties. Individual Gm antigens are only associated with one particular IgG subclass. In IgG1, which is the major subclass, Gm(a) and Gm(f) function as allelic markers. When the series of Gm markers available for IgG1, IgG2 and IgG3 heavy chain genes are analyzed in families, it is apparent that they are closely linked.[6] The region of the chromosome governing λ, a and possibly μ chains can be pictured (Fig. 1) as a series of closely positioned loci numbering from 4 to perhaps as many as 15 or 20. Without going into greater detail, a genetic marker, Am(2+), has been localized to IgA heavy chains and found to segregate in association with the Gm markers demonstrating linkage.[7] Animal studies in comparable Ig allotypic systems predict that all heavy chain constant region genes will be localized to the same chromosomal region. The linkage group of Gm genes for human λ heavy chains has been referred to as a Gm gene complex.[6]

Genetic defects in Gm structural genes have been searched for by using knowledge of the constitution of Gm gene complexes in different populations. In one family there is evidence for genetic transmission of a Gm gene complex lacking an IgG1 gene (Table 2).[8] In the sera II3 and II6, Gm(b) is found in individuals who are negative for Gm(f). This is highly unusual in Caucasian sera since these two antigens are usually present together in the same Gm gene complex. An alternative explanation is the presence of a rare gene complex in which Gm(b) is associated with Gm(a) rather than

14

TABLE 1

Sub Classes of IgG Heavy Chains

Subclass	%	Gm Markers	Phenotypes		
IgG1	70	(a)	a/a	a/f	f/f
		(f)			
IgG2	18	(n)			
IgG3	8	(b)	b/b	b/g	g/g
		(g)			
IgG4	3				

HEAVY CHAIN GENE COMPLEXES

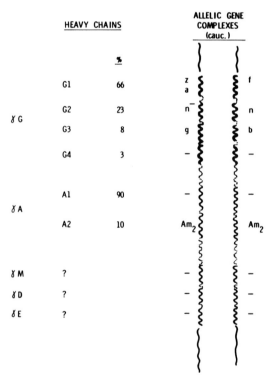

Fig. 1. Schematic representation of chromosomal region and gene loci for human Ig heavy chains. The alphabetical letters refer to *Gm* genes. The % of IgG and IgA, composed of each subclass respectively, are given.

TABLE 2

Sera Allotype Concentrations in a Family Carrying a *Gm*
Gene Complex Lacking an *IgG1* Gene*

Sera		Presumed Gm Gene type	Gm (f)	mg/ml in sera Gm (a)	IgG
II	3	*b,−/g, a*	0	6.40	11.33
II	6	*b,−/g, a*	0	5.97	12.38
III	4	*b,−/b, f*	5.40	0	12.76
III	5	*b,−/b, f*	5.60	0	9.41
NORMALS					
Heterozygotes			3.52	2.99	
Homozygotes			6.70	5.28	

*The − in the genotype refers to the presumably absent *IgG1 Gm* gene.

17

Gm(f). This was excluded by pedigree analysis of the third generation in which the aberrant gene complex was present in conjunction with a gene complex lacking Gm(a).[8] It was concluded from more complete data, not presented here, that this family inherited a segregating gene complex for Ig heavy chains that lacked a Gm gene coding for any known IgG1 marker. Quantitative studies strongly suggested that the IgG1 gene was absent from the aberrant gene complex rather than "silent".[8]

The segregation of a gene complex with a missing *IgG1* gene provided insight into the control of Ig synthesis by the remaining normal *IgG1* gene present in heterozygous carriers of the unusual gene complex. The individuals with the aberrant *Gm* gene complex had Gm allotype concentrations similar to normal homozygous controls, suggesting dosage compensation for the missing allele appears to be operative (Table 2). A similar phenomenon has been described in rabbits[9] and in mice.[10]

In summary, structural Ig genes detected by Gm antigenic markers on γ heavy chains can be localized to specific amino acids and their genetic transmission analyzed in families. Genetically stable deletions of allotype genes have been demonstrated at low incidence in human populations. Mechanisms exist which compensate for the dosage effect in some families.

II. *Immune response (Ir) genes* are genes controlling inherited differences in immune response to *specific antigens* as delineated by experimental studies in strains of mice and guinea pigs. The differences between responder and non-responder strains are, in general, quantitative. Non-responder animals produce antibody of appropriate specificity although predominantly or solely of IgM class[11] and differ from responder animals in the level of the response. It has not been ruled out that non-responder animals may produce antibodies of slightly different primary structure although of similar specificity.

The biological properties of Ir genes can be compared to the Gm structural genes of man (Table 3). Present evidence indicates that the responder trait is antigen specific and controlled by a single autosomal dominant gene affected by modifiers. Studies in several laboratories show that Ir genes are expressed in T lymphocytes in contrast to structural allotype genes which operate, to the best of our present knowledge, in the antibody synthesizing B lymphocyte. One critical aspect of the Ir genes is their close linkage to genes defining the major histocompatibility loci.[12] In autosomal dominant or co-dominant genes, the biologic differences in specificity, mediated by different populations of lymphocytes and the genetic differences in linkage sharply distinguish them.

Ir genes, to date, have been described in laboratory animals. Levine and co-workers, however, have reported recently that there are differences in the

TABLE 3

Biologic Properties of *Gm* and *Ir* Genes

	Gm	*Ir*
Genetic Control	AUTOSOMAL DOMINANT UNIGENIC	+
Specificity	MULTIPLE ANTIGENS	ONE ANTIGEN
Lymphocyte	B CELL	T CELL
Linkage	ONLY A1AT*	HISTO-INCOMPATIBILITY LOCI
Gene Product	HEAVY CHAIN	? SURFACE RECEPTOR OF T CELLS

+*Gm* genes are co-dominant; *Ir* genes dominant.

*α-1-antitrypsin.

level of the immune response of the IgE antibody to ragweed pollen in man.[13]

III. All discussions involving *control genes* for Igs are less clear and more conjectural than the description of structural and immune response genes. Although evidence for the existence of regulatory genes in microorganisms has been carefully detailed in recent years, in eukaryotes most of the evidence remains inferential. I shall discuss selected examples, some from our own studies, which suggest the operation of regulatory genetic mechanisms for Ig.

a. It appears that quantitative regulation of the immune response can occur at the level of the Gm gene complex. In our laboratory[14] and that of Morell *et al.*[15] differences in IgG subclass concentrations in serum have been demonstrated in groups of subjects differing in allotypic *Gm* genes. Among the most striking examples are the two to three-fold higher concentrations of IgG3 subclass[16] and genetic antigen[14] in the serum of persons with *Gm(b)* as compared to the allelic *Gm(g)* gene. In the case of IgG1 heavy chains, *Gm(f)* appears to result in higher allotype concentrations than *Gm(a)*;[17] an analogous situation may be present for *Gm^n* as compared to persons lacking this gene.[17] It should be noted that all of the Gm genes associated with higher allotype values, i.e. *Gm^b, Gm f, Gm^n* are in a *cis* position with respect to each other. The *Gm* gene complex may be critical in the determination of the levels of immune response, perhaps, because of cis linkage to a limited pool of variable region genes.

b. Click and co-workers have demonstrated that the *in vitro* response (plaque forming cells) of inbred strains of mice to sheep red blood cells were, in many cases, greater than the *in vivo* response.[18] The differences were genetically determined. They concluded, in further experiments, that at least two genes were involved, one of them regulating the magnitude of the response. The above systems were complex and differed from the *Gm* and *Ir* genes in being dependent on gene dosage (hybrids had intermediate results). Similar biologic mechanisms may explain the data of Biozzi *et al.*[19] who showed parallel genetic segregation of the immune response to unrelated antigens in Swiss mice selectively bred for their responses to sheep and pigeon red cells.

c. Perhaps the most compelling body of evidence available on the existence of control genes has been obtained from study of immune states in man. Several facts imply the existence of regulatory genes for Igs: 1) A considerable number of the inherited immunodeficiencies are X-linked. However, the known structural and *Ir* genes for *Ig* are autosomal. The nature of the genetic controls mediated by genes on the X-chromosome is unclear, nor is it known whether there is random inactivation of one chromosome early in development as there is for the X-chromosome. 2) The mutant genes involved in the X-linked immunodeficiencies and other humoral immunodeficiencies are quantitative, i.e. they result in low but not absent Igs. The Igs remaining in affected persons appear, by present antigenic and immunochemical criteria, similar to Ig found in normal sera. Although this quantitative feature resembles the activity of *Ir* genes, human immunodeficiencies are not antigen specific as are *Ir* genes. 3) Selective allotypic depressions are found in families with variable immuno-deficiencies. This phenomenon implies genetic determination of these disorders by dominant genes regulating allotype Ig synthesis but which appear to differ from the structural *Gm* genes described above.[20]

I would like to conclude this overview with the conjecture that inter-relationships between regulatory and structural genes are also involved in immune deficiency diseases. The above phenomenon was brought to attention by the description of the Hx family.[21] A family in which there was evidence for a deleted IgG1 Gm gene, has been described in Table 2. Three of 4 selected families studied had similar findings, including compensatory synthesis.[8] In one family, however, the carriers of the aberrant gene had reduced concentrations of IgG; one also had low IgA and IgM. The failure of dosage compensation may have contributed to development of an immunodeficiency state in this last family. These data raise a question concerning the circumstances which allow interaction between structural gene defects and regulatory mechanisms to result in clinical disorders.

Data on current approaches to genetic control of Ig have been received in terms of *structural, immune response* and *control genes*. The degree of progress on the above problems is apparent from an increasing ability to interrelate experimentally described genetic controls with defects of the immune response in man.

REFERENCES

1. H.O. McDevitt and M. Landy, Genetic Control of Immune Responsiveness, Academic Press, New York, London, 1972.

2. R. Grubb, The Genetic Markers of Human Immunoglobulins, Springer-Verlag, New York and Heidelberg, 1970.

3. S.D. Litwin and H.G. Kunkel, *J. Exper. Med. 125,* 847, 1967.

4. R. Mage, *in* Progress in Immunology, 1st Inter. Congr. Immun., B. Amos (Ed.), Academic Press, 47, 1971.

5. T. Gedde-Dahl, M.K. Fagerhal, P.J.L. Cook and J. Noades, *J. Ann. Hum. Genet. 35,* 393, 1972.

6. J.B. Natvig, H.G. Kunkel and S.D. Litwin, *Cold Spring Harbor Symp. Quant. Biol. 32,* 173, 1967.

7. H.G. Kunkel, W.K. Smith, F.G. Joslin, J.B. Natvig and S.D. Litwin, *Nature 223,* 1247, 1969.

8. S.D. Litwin, *in* Proc. 4th Inter. Cong. Hum. Genet., Paris, Excerpta Medica (Amst.), Int. Congr. Series No. 233, 113, 1971.

9. R.G. Mage, *Symp. Quant. Biol. 32,* 203, 1967.

10. E.B. Jacobsen, L.A. Herzenberg, R. Riblet and L.A. Herzenberg, *J. Exper. Med. 135,* 1151, 1972.

11. F.C. Grumet, *Fed. Proc. 30,* 469, 1971.

12. B. Benacerraf and H.O. McDevitt, *Science 175,* 273, 1972.

13. B.B. Levine, R. Stember and M. Fotino, *Science 178,* 1201, 1972.

14. S.D. Litwin, *J. Immunol. 106,* 589, 1971.

15. A. Morell, F. Skvaril, A.G. Steinberg, E. van Loghem and W.D. Terry, *J. Immunol. 108,* 195, 1972.

16. W.J. Yount, H.G. Kunkel and S.D. Litwin, *J. Exper. Med. 125,* 177, 1967.

17. A.G. Steinberg, A. Morell, F. Skvaril and E. van Loghem, *J. Immunol. 110,* 1642, 1973.

18. R.E. Click, L. Benck, B.J. Alter and J.C. Lovchik, *J. Exper. Med. 136,* 1241, 1972.

19. G. Biozzi, R. Asofsky, R. Lieberman, C. Stiffel, D. Mouton and B. Benacerraf, *J. Exper. Med. 132,* 752, 1970.

20. S.D. Litwin and H.H. Fudenberg, Proc. Nat. Acad. Sci. USA, Vol. 69, No. 7, 1739, 1972.

21. W.J. Yount, R. Hong, M. Seligman, R. Good and H.G. Kunkel, *J. Clin. Invest. 49,* 1957, 1966.

AUTHOR'S NOTE

Abbreviations: IgG, immunoglobulin G; IgG1, immunoglobulin G1; IgG2, immunoglobulin G2; IgG3, immunoglobulin G3; IgG4, immunoglobulin G4; Gm factors, genetic antigens of human immunoglobulin G.

Human sera contain four IgG subclasses (IgG1, IgG2, IgG3, IgG4). Gm(a) and Gm(f) are Gm genetic factors for antithetical structural genes for IgG1 heavy chains. Gm(g) and Gm(b) are similarly Gm markers for antithetical genes of IgG3 chains. The numerical designation for the Gm antigens is as follows: Gm(a) = (1); Gm(f) = (4); Gm(g) = (21); Gm(b) = (5); Gm(z) = (17).

HETEROGENEITY OF THE IMMUNODEFICIENCY SYNDROMES*

Fred S. Rosen

Immunity results from many interacting mechanisms which may be specific or nonspecific. The failure of one or another *specific* immunity mechanisms results in immunodeficiency disease. It has been known for two decades that there is a clear-cut dichotomy between cellular and humoral immunity. This division of labor in the immune response has a cellular basis and recently methods have been developed to identify the various lymphoidal cells which are responsible for humoral or cellular immunity. Those lymphocytes which mediate cellular immunity are called T lymphocytes because they are thymus-dependent for their competence. Cells which differentiate to synthesize and secrete immunoglobulins are designated B cells, as they are derived from the bone marrow or bursa of Fabricus in avian species. Immunodeficiencies may be classified according to their B or T cell deficits or both[1] (Table 1).

PRIMARY B CELL DEFICIENCIES

The outstanding clinical manifestation of patients with quantitative or qualitative defects of B cell function is recurrent, invasive infection with pyogenic bacteria. These infections are not different from those observed in normal individuals of the same age — pyoderma, pharyngitis, sinusitis, otitis media, pneumonia, sepsis and meningitis. They respond normally to antibiotics but are notable for their frequency and often for their severity. There is a diminished or absent antibody response to injected antigens or to infection, which has given rise to the term introduced by the Swiss workers — the *antibody deficiency syndrome.* Since this basic pathogenetic defect results in failure of phagocytosis, an essential step in the control of invasion by pyogenic bacteria, it is not surprising that an indistinguishable clinical picture has been observed in patients with deficiency of the third component or complement (C3). Cellular immune responses of the T cells

*Supported by USPHS grant AI-05877-11.

TABLE 1

PRIMARY IMMUNODEFICIENCIES

Type	Suggested Cellular Defect			Inheritance		
	B cells Circulating Ig-bearing B lymphocytes (a)*	B lymphocytes (b)**	T cells	X-linked	Autosomal Recessive	Other†
X-linked agammaglobulinemia	X	(X)††		X		
Thymic hypoplasia			X			X
Severe combined immunodeficiency	X	(X)	X	X	X	X
with dysostosis	X	?	X		X	
with adenosine deaminase deficiency	X		X		X	
with generalized hemopoietic hypoplasia	X		X		X.	
Selective Ig deficiency						
IgA	?	X	(X)			X
Others	?	?				X
X-linked immunodeficiencies with inc. M	X	X		X		
Immunodeficiency with ataxia telangiectasia	X	X	X		X?	
Immunodeficiency with thrombocytopenia and eczema (**W**iskott-Aldrich syndrome)			X	X		
Immunodeficiency with thymoma	X*		X			X
Immunodeficiency with normo- or hyper-gammaglobulinemia	X	X	(X)		X	X
Transient hypogammaglobulinemia of infancy	X	X			X	X
Varied immunodeficiencies (largely unclassified and common)	X	X	(X)		(X)	X

*Absent or very low

**Easily detectable or increased

†Implies multifactorial or unknown genetic basis or no genetic basis

††Some cases with circulating B lymphocytes without detectable surface Ig have been found

being preserved, these patients respond to most viral, fungal or mycobacterial infections normally. A number of different primary disorders can give rise to the antibody deficiency syndrome.

Transient Hypogammaglobulinemia of Infancy

Normally, the synthesis of immunoglobulins in response to infection and other antigenic stimuli begins after birth. However, if the fetus is infected *in utero* after the 20th week of gestation by rubella virus, cytomegalovirus, *Toxoplasma* or syphilis, he (or she) can mount an impressive antibody response to the invasive pathogen. This antibody response, consisting largely of IgM and to a lesser extent of IgA and IgG antibodies, can be helpful in the diagnosis of prenatal infection. A cord or neonatal serum level of IgM in excess of 20 mg per 100 ml is considered presumptive evidence of intra-uterine infection.[2] The level of IgG, which is passively acquired by transplacental passage, falls rapidly during the first month of life, levels off during the second month and soon begins to rise. Rarely, there is delay in the maturation of B cells and their immunologic function; the level of IgG globulins received by passive transfer from the mother continues to fall and is not adequately raised by immunoglobulins synthesized by the infant, so that within a few months the total gammaglobulin level is much lower than usual for that age. The infants have overt infections, unexplained episodes of fever and often bronchitis with wheezing. Regular injections of gammaglobulin will protect them from severe, invasive infections. The injections may be discontinued when the IgG globulins begin to rise toward normal levels, usually before the age of 3 years. The cause of this transient hypogamma-globulinemia is not known. Normal numbers of B cells are present in the circulation of affected infants.

X-linked Agammaglobulinemia
(Congenital Agammaglobulinemia; Bruton's Disease)

X-linked agammaglobulinemia usually manifests itself in the second year of life, although onset of the characteristically severe recurrent infections may begin at any age from 8 months to 3 years. The infections are those caused by the common pyogenic organisms — *Staphylococcus aureus,* pneumococci, meningococci, *Hemophilus influenzae* and, less often, beta-hemolytic strepto-cocci or *Pseudomonas.* They differ from infections in normal children only in their frequency, severity and the tendency for infection with the same organism to occur more than once. Pyoderma, purulent conjunctivitis, pharyngitis, otitis media, sinusitis, bronchitis, pneumonia, empyema, purulent arthritis, meningitis and sepsis occur with surprising frequency and may be associated with unusually high fever and unexpected elevation or depression of the leukocyte count. A rather indolent rheumatoid-like arthritis with sterile effusion into one of the large joints develops in about one-third of patients and may be the presenting complaint. The children usually, but not always, handle most viral infections normally.[3]

There should be a high index of suspicion about this diagnosis on the basis of the history of repeated severe bacterial infections. A careful family history may uncover instances of death from overwhelming infection or multiple severe infections in other brothers, maternal uncles or sons of maternal aunts. Examination reveals little except the signs of infection, evidence of joint involvement if present and usually small, smooth tonsils. Lateral films of the pharynx fail to reveal an adenoid shadow. Lymph nodes are small but palpable; regional nodes may be swollen and tender during episodes of infection. Immunochemical assay reveals a marked diminution of IgM, IgA and IgG globulins in the serum. It is important to remember that, because of individual variations and the low levels of immunoglobulins normally found in the early months of life, the diagnosis cannot be firmly established by immunoelectrophoresis until 6 to 8 months of age. However, failure of IgM or IgA to appear in significant concentration and a steady fall in IgG during the first 3 to 4 months of life should suggest the diagnosis, especially in the presence of a positive family history. Isohemagglutinins are usually absent or in very low titer. Injections of vaccines is not followed by an adequate antibody rise and removal of a stimulated regional lymph node discloses absence of the expected germinal centers, secondary follicles and plasma cells.

The thymus is normal but lymph nodes and spleen lack the usual follicular architecture. Germinal centers are absent and there are few if any plasma cells in the medullary cores or red pulp. Although the number of lymphocytes in the tissues appears diminished, they are present in the thymus-dependent areas of lymphoid tissue and normal numbers are found in the blood. Plasma cells are absent from the bone marrow. Plasma cells, however, may be normally absent from the bone marrow in children under 5 years of age, so that this is not a helpful finding.[19] Study of the circulating lymphocytes has revealed normal numbers of T cells but complete absence of B cells. We have found normal numbers of B cells in only one case of proved X-linked agammaglobulinemia These B cells are abnormal in that they are unresponsive to the T cell mitogen and pokeweed mitogen and do not synthesize immunoglobulins *in vitro.*

Provided the diagnosis is made before repeated infections have produced anatomic damage (e.g., bronchiectasis, pulmonary insufficiency, middle ear deafness), the immediate prognosis for these children is excellent and they gain and grow normally. In later childhood, adolescence or early adult life, however, complications may develop in some of these patients. Slowly progressive neurologic disease, suggesting a "slow virus" infection, may accompany a dermatomyositis-like syndrome with brawny edema, perivascular mononuclear infiltrates and, terminally, severe systemic symptoms and death. Thus far, no consistent cause for these complications has been found. An enterovirus was repeatedly isolated from blood, stool and spinal fluid in the last patient to succumb with the dermatomyositis-like picture.

X-linked Immunodeficiency with Increased IgM

In a few instances, patients are observed with manifestations similar to those in X-linked agammaglobulinemia but with higher levels of immuno-globulins which, when analyzed, turn out to reflect a marked deficiency of serum IgA and IgG but an elevation in the concentration of IgM. The congenital form of this disease seems to occur almost entirely in males and has a suggestive X-linked pattern of inheritance. Except for a greater frequency of "autoimmune" hematologic disorders (neutropenia, hemolytic anemia, thrombocytopenia), the clinical course in these patients resembles that of X-linked agammaglobulinemia.[5] Histologically, there is disorganization of the follicular architecture of the lymphoid tissues, but PAS-positive plasmacytoid cells containing IgM are present and even tonsillar hypertrophy due to these cells has been observed. Only B cells with IgM surface fluorescence are found. No B cells with surface IgA or IgG are present. Similar disturbances of the immunoglobulin picture associated with the antibody deficiency syndrome have been seen in adults with frequent respiratory tract infections and bronchiectasis and in some infants with congenital rubella.

Selective Immunoglobulin Deficiencies
(Dysgammaglobulinemia)

This term is used to describe cases in which there are consistent deficiencies of one or more of the recognizable plasma immunoglobulins. Although often associated with the clinical manifestations of the antibody deficiency syndrome, some instances of selective immunoglobulin deficiency may be chance laboratory findings in otherwise apparently normal individuals.

Selective deficiency of IgG subclasses may occur, in which the patient is unable to synthesize one or more of the IgG subclasses and thus fails to produce antibodies in one or more of the four presently identified IgG subclasses. This results in failure to respond to particular types of antigens, in increased susceptibility to a limited spectrum of bacterial infections and in a reduction of total serum IgG concentration proportional to the percentage of the total IgG pool accounted for by the deficient IgG subclass. Of course, a deficiency in IgG1 is most severe, since this subclass constitutes over 70% of

29

of the IgG.[6,7]

Selective IgA deficiency is observed with considerable frequency (3 to 7 per 1000 population). In a few patients, this may portend the development of ataxia telangiectasia but an appreciable number of such individuals remain healthy throughout life. However, a high incidence of rheumatoid arthritis, systemic lupus erythematosus and malabsorption syndrome has been observed among this group of patients.[8,9] A significant number of IgA-deficient individuals have circulating antibodies to IgA and have anaphylactic reactions upon receiving whole blood or plasma.[10]

Deficiency of secretory IgA may well play a role in undue susceptibility to certain infections, particularly viral, of the respiratory and gastrointestinal tracts. Secretory IgA is the form of antibody synthesized in plasma cells closely related to the mucous membranes and secreted into colostrum, saliva and respiratory and intestinal secretions as two subunits of IgA in combination with a "secretory piece" synthesized by the epithelial cells and another polypeptide chain which stabilizes the polymer (J chain). Thus, deficiency of this type of local immunity may contribute to the clinical picture of agammaglobulinemia and ataxia telangiectasia, as well as to the tendency to recurrent otitis media or to chronic diarrhea in some patients with selective IgA deficiency. Likewise, the efficacy of certain respiratory viral vaccines when administered intranasally or of oral poliomyelitis vaccine may depend more upon the establishment of local immunity than upon the stimulation of systemic antibody formation.[11] It is difficult to assess "secretory" immunity.

Rare cases of *immunodeficiency with normal or increased immunoglobulins* have been observed, in which the classic picture of the antibody deficiency syndrome was accompanied by a normal or even increased level of immunoglobulins and the presence of plasma cells in the tissues but a failure to form specific antibodies to a variety of antigens. These have not been adequately studied with modern methods to provide an adequate explanation.[12]

Variable Unclassified Immunodeficiency (Dysgammaglobulinemia)

This is the most common form of immunodeficiency with serious clinical consequences and probably includes a number of entities; it occurs in either sex at any age without any known causative factor, either genetic or acquired, although a predisposition may be inherited since its development has been reported in siblings or among relatives.

The picture is that of the antibody deficiency syndrome associated with immunoglobulin deficiency, which may be somewhat less severe than in the X-linked form of agammaglobulinemia. Pathologically, there is necrobiotic change in the follicular architecture of the lymph nodes and spleen or lymphadenopathy and splenomegaly due to reticulum cell hyperplasia. The predominant infections are sinusitis and pneumonia, often leading to bronchiectasis unless intensively treated. Although the rheumatoid arthritis-like complications are occasionally seen, a sprue-like malabsorption syndrome and pernicious anemia are more common. Recent work has demonstrated that this malabsorption syndrome is often due to *Giardia lamblia* demonstrated either in aspirates of duodenal fouid or in biopsy specimens of duodenal mucosa.[13]

Management is the same as for X-linked agammaglobulinemia: substitution therapy with regular injections of large doses of immune serum globulin for prophylaxis and intensive antimicrobial therapy for acute infections. The chronic diarrhea and malabsorption due to giardiasis, which may give a picture of protein-losing enteropathy, usually respond promptly to metronidazole (Flagyl) in doses of 0.25 g t.i.d. for five days.

Patients with "acquired" agammaglobulinemia may have no B cells but, more commonly, normal numbers of B cells or even increased numbers of B cells do not synthesize immunoglobulin; in others, immunoglobulin synthesis is normal but there is no secretion of the immunoglobulin formed. We have studied one patient whose B cells functioned normally *in vitro* when cultured in normal AB+ serum but did not in the patient's serum. Obviously a whole spectrum of B cell maturation failure is presented by these patients. T cell function deteriorates progressively. This is particularly true of patients who have an associated thyoma.

PRIMARY T CELL DEFICIENCIES

Patients with T cell deficiency have much more serious susceptibility to infection than patients with complete or partial B cell defects. In its most severe forms, T cell deficiency results in an inability to terminate opportunistic infections with organisms that are ordinarily innocuous. Consequently, varicella, vaccinia, herpes and measles viruses can be fatal infections. The enterobacilli are invasive and infection with *Monilia* is common. Malignancy of both the lymphoreticular organs and other viscera is also a common complication of the T cell disorders.

Severe Combined Immunodeficiency

Severe combined immunodeficiency (Swiss type agammaglobulinemia, alymphocytosis, thymic alymphoplasia) is the most profound of the cellular defects. Affected patients usually have no T or B cells; the disease is invariably fatal. It is genetically determined and there is clear evidence of autosomal recessive and X-linked recessive transmission of the disease. The clinical and

31

laboratory findings may be quite variable from case to case, even among affected members of a single family.

The onset of persistent infection of the lungs, monilial infection of the oropharynx, esophagus and skin, chronic diarrhea, and wasting and runting begins in the early months of life and progresses with monotonous regularity to a fatal termination despite all attempts at routine therapy. Affected infants usually do not survive the first year or two of life. Examination usually reveals absence of tonsils, very small or absent lymph nodes despite chronic infection, chronic pneumonitis evidenced by a pertussis-like cough, inspiratory retractions of the chest, rales, a somewhat distended abdomen with wasting and oral thrush.[15]

Roentgenographic signs include pulmonary infiltrations and absence of a thymic shadow. There is usually an absolute decrease in the number of circulating lymphocytes and occasionally neutropenia. In typical cases, the immunoglobulins are markedly decreased but variants have been described in which circulating immunoglobulins are normal or there is selective immunoglobulin deficiency. M components may be present in the circulation.[16] Plasma cells have been found in the tissues of such patients but antibody formation is almost always impaired or absent. Tests of delayed hypersensitivity give negative results: sensitization cannot be induced with dinitrochlorobenzene, cultured lymphocytes do not respond to phytohemagglutinin and skin allografts are not rejected. T cells are almost always absent from the circulation and the few lymphocytes present in the blood usually have the characteristics of B cells.

Treatment of the infections in these patients must be specific. Pulmonary infection is frequently due to *Pneumocystis carini,* requiring pentamidine or pyrimethamine and sulfadiazine. Routine antimicrobial therapy, fungistatic drugs or human gammaglobulin are only temporarily effective and do not prevent the inexorable, fatal course of the disease if the immunologic deficiency is not overcome. The use of attenuated viral or BCG vaccines must be avoided, since the attenuated viruses or mycobacteria can produce fatal generalized disease and natural infection with herpes, varicella or measles is uniformly and progressively fatal.

The establishment of immunologic competence with transplants of bone marrow in these infants is still experimental and should only be carried out in those centers with adequate manpower, clinical and laboratory experience and physical facilities for what is an exacting ordeal for patient, family, nurses and physicians. Success depends upon attention to a number of factors.[17−20]

For an index case in a family, the diagnosis is seldom made until infection is already established. Every subsequent sibling should be carefully watched for early signs of the disease — absence of clinically demonstrable thymic tissue at birth, low peripheral lymphocyte count, absence of serum IgM and IgA and failure of cultured lymphocytes from cord blood or subsequent blood samples to respond to phytohemagglutinin. Affected infants can be maintained in a sterile environment or laminar flow apparatus with exquisite care in administration of systemic and topical antibiotics.

A donor of bone marrow whose cells are HL-A identical and can be shown to be histocompatible *in vitro* by mixed lymphocyte culture (MLC) should be identified. In practice, this almost always means a sibling. However, a successful transplant from an MLC-identical maternal uncle has been accomplished despite HL-A non-identity between donor and recipient. Administration of a suitable dose of bone marrow cells from the donor when the infant is as free of infection as possible is accomplished with 50×10^6 nucleated cells per kilo I.V. More cells are optimal to I.P. injection, perhaps 50×10^7. Evidence that the graft has become established and that immunologic reconstitution (T cell function as shown by phytohemagglutinin responses, B cell function by immunoglobulin synthesis) has occurred usually requires three to eight weeks.

In skilled hands, patients with this hitherto fatal disease have been cured and appear normal. Nevertheless, success is not universal, there is much to learn and the treatment is heroic. Intrauterine diagnosis of this disorder has not been accomplished but might ultimately lead to its prevention in affected families. The possibility of finding ADA deficiency in amnion cells remains to be explored.

Variant forms of severe combined immunodeficiency have been described. These include cases with dysostosis (short-limbed dwarfism) and rare cases with generalized hemopoietic hypoplasia. The latter has been called reticular dysgenesis; infants with this type of immunodeficiency also lack granulocytic precursors in the bone marrow and granulocytes in peripheral blood and survive for only a short time after birth.[21] Nezelof syndrome, which is severe combined immunodeficiency with normal immunoglobulins, is a specious diagnosis and the term should be dropped. This variant is included in the term severe combined immunodeficiency.

Immunodeficiency with Ataxia Telangiectasia

This is an autosomal recessive disease in which abnormalities of the thymus have been found postmortem. Gradually progressive cerebellar ataxia begins in early childhood. This is associated with increasing telangiectasia, which first becomes apparent as a rather inconspicuous dilatation of small blood vessels in the bulbar conjunctivae and ultimately is visible in the skin at about 5 years of age. Gonadal dysgenesis and failure of sexual maturation may be present in those who survive into the second decade.

In late childhood, recurrent sinobronchial infections begin in many patients, often leading to bronchiectasis. There is also a tendency to the development of malignant tumors, particularly of the lymphoid system. These reflect an immunologic disturbance affecting T cell function, as shown by blunting of delayed hypersensitivity reactions, failure to reject allografts normally and delayed response of the lymphocytes to phytohemagglutinin. At postmortem examination late in the disease, the thymus is abnormally small and has a decreased number of lymphocytes; there is a poor differentiation between cortex and medulla and decided diminution in Hassall's corpuscles. The number of circulating lymphocytes and the architecture of the lymph nodes vary considerably and do not always correlate well with the patient's history. The most consistent B cell defect is a low level or absence of IgA globulin in the serum, which occurs in about 70% of affected persons and may precede clinical evidence of immunologic deficiency by a number of years.[22]

Immunodeficiency with Thrombocytopenia and Eczema (Wiskott-Aldrich Syndrome)

The Wiskott-Aldrich syndrome is an X-linked recessive disorder which is usually manifested by eczema, thrombocytopenia and a wide variety of infections beginning late in the first year, although it may present rarely as thrombocytopenia alone. Death may occur from hemorrhage, infection or the development of a malignant process similar to the Letterer-Siwe type of reticuloendotheliosis.

The infections may be caused by a wide variety of microorganisms, including viruses, bacteria, fungi and *Pneumocystis carinii.* Transient episodes of arthritis have been observed.

Results of studies of the pathogenesis of the Wiskott-Aldrich syndrome are confusing. The lymphoid tissues appear normal early in the course of the disease but as it progresses there may be a loss of lymphocytes from the thymus and paracortical areas of the lymph nodes. The peripheral lymphocyte count may decrease and there is a variable loss of cellular immunity, resulting in increased susceptibility to viral of fungal disease. Studies of immunoglobulin production in these patients suggest normal responses to a variety of antigens. IgM values are often low and isohemagglutinins and Forssman antibodies, normally present as "natural" antibodies, are usually lacking. The failure of these patients to respond to pneumococcal polysaccharides has led to the postulation that they have a general inability to respond to polysaccharide antigens, as opposed to normal responses to protein antigens.[23, 24] Whether this failure resides in the recognition system of the lymphocytes, in a deficit of the macrophages in processing such antigens or in a qualitative deficiency of plasma cell function is not clear. Since polysaccharides are widely distributed and important constituents of bacteria and fungi, it is reasonable that such a selective immunologic deficiency might have a serious impact upon resistance. Transfer factor has been tried and found to induce cellular immunity and clinical improvement in some patients with this disease.[29]

Congenital Thymic Aplasia
(DiGeorge Syndrome)

Congenital thymic aplasia (DiGeorge syndrome, third and fourth pharyngeal pouch syndrome) results from a failure of the normal embryogenesis of the thymus and parathyroid glands, which are derived from the third and fourth pharyngeal clefts. The syndrome is not genetically determined but appears rather to result from some intrauterine accident before the eighth week of gestation. Affected infants invariably have neonatal tetany. Anomalies of the great blood vessels are very frequently encountered, usually right-sided aortic arch, as is tetralogy of Fallot.[28] These cardiac complications are the cause of late death in these children.[26] Mental subnormality also accompanies this syndrome.

The T cell defect in children with congenital thymic aplasia varies from the most profound to the barely discernible. In any case, T cell function improves in these children with age, so that by 5 years of age no T cell deficit can be ascertained. It is not clear how this grossly retarded T cell maturation occurs in the absence of a thymus gland. Some children may have a small thymic remnant but T cell maturation may occur at sites other than the thymus.

Transplants of fetal thymus into these infants results in a rapid acquisition of T cell function.[27,28] A hormone-like substance is thought to be secreted by the thymic epithelium. It has been called "thymosin" and it is presumed to effect T cell maturation.[29] It has thus far eluded isolation.

SUMMARY

The foregoing discussion has included those immunodeficiency syndromes into which patients can be readily classified. A vast reservoir of patients with unclassifiable defects exists. Even within these clear-cut syndromes, there is great variability in the clinical course, the laboratory abnormalities and even genetic transmission and penetrance. Much work remains to be done to clarify the various etiologies of immunodeficiency.

REFERENCES

1. WHO Committee, *Pediatrics 47,* 927, 1971.

2. C.A. Alford, J. Schaefer *et al., New Engl. J. Med. 277,* 437, 1967.

3. F.S. Rosen and C.A. Janeway, *J. Pediat. 68,* 652, 1966.

4. R.S. Geha, F.S. Rosen *et al., J. Clin. Invest. 52,* 1725, 1973.

5. F.S. Rosen, S.V. Kevy *et al., Pediatrics 28,* 182, 1961.

6. P. Schur, H. Borel *et al., New Engl. J. Med. 283,* 631, 1970.

7. W.S. Yount, R. Hong *et al., J. Clin. Invest. 49,* 1957, 1970.

8. P. A. Crabbe and J.F. Heremans, *Am. J. Med. 42,* 319, 1967.

9. A.J. Ammann and R. Hong, *Clin. Exp. Immunol. 7,* 833, 1970.

10. G.N. Vyas, H.A. Perkins *et al., Lancet 2,* 312, 1968.

11. P.L. Ogra, D.T. Karzan *et al., New Engl. J. Med. 279,* 893, 1968.

12. A. Giedion and J.J. Scheidegger, *Helv. Pediatr. Acta 12,* 241, 1957.

13. H.D. Ochs, M.E. Ament *et al., New Engl. J. Med. 287,* 341, 1972.

14. R. Geha, E. Schneeberger *et al., New Engl. J. Med.,* 1974 (in press).

15. F.S. Rosen and C.A. Janeway, *New Engl. J. Med. 275,* 769, 1966.

16. R.S. Geha, E. Schneeberger *et al., New Engl. J. Med.,* 1974 (in press).

17. R.A. Gatti, H.J. Meuwissen *et al., Lancet 2,* 1366, 1968.

18. J. deKoning, D.W. van Bekkum *et al., Lancet 1,* 1223, 1969.

19. R.H. Levey, E.W. Gelfand *et al., Lancet 2,* 571, 1971.

20. M.E. Stiehm, G.J. Lawlor, Jr. *et al., New Engl. J. Med. 286,* 797, 1972.

21. D. Gitlin, G. Vawter *et al., Pediatrics 33,* 184, 1964.

22. R.D.A. Peterson, W.D. Kelly *et al., Lancet 1,* 1189, 1964.

23. R.M. Blaese, R.S. Brown *et al., Lancet 1,* 1056, 1968.

24. M.D. Cooper, H.P. Chase *et al., Am. J. Med. 44,* 499, 1968.

25. A.M. DiGeorge, *Birth Defects Orig. Art. Ser. 4,* 116, 1968.

26. R.M. Freedom, F.S. Rosen *et al., Circulation 16,* 165, 1972.

27. C.S. August, F.S. Rosen *et al., Lancet 2,* 1210, 1968.

28. W.W. Cleveland, B.J. Fogel *et al., Lancet 2,* 1211, 1968.

29. A.L. Goldstein, A. Guha *et al., Proc. Natl. Acad. Sci. USA 69,* 1800, 1972.

DISCUSSION

DR. PORTER: Dr. Litwin, you say that as the gammaglobulins are determined by autosomal structural genes and as the immune deficiency states are X-linked, the latter may be controlled by regulator genes. I do not understand how you come to this conclusion. After all, the gammaglobulins may not be the primary gene products in the immune deficiency states.

DR. LITWIN: I have used the term regulatory gene in a broad sense to refer to any genes which affect immune response but which differ from both the structural immunoglobulin genes for which we have allotypic markers (Gm and Inv) and the immune response genes linked to histocompatibility antigens. These genetic controls may not be similar to the operator or regulator genes described for the lactose operon of *E. coli:* they may specify gene products as Dr. Porter points out, which indirectly influence immunoglobulin production.

RALPH FREDMAN (Wassaic State School, Wassaic, New York): I would like to ask a question concerning *in vivo* and *in vitro* immunoglobulins in the lymphocytes. *In vivo* there were none and *in vitro* there were immunoglobulins. What happens in the cultured cell that doesn't happen in the body? In the cultured cell you get immunoglobulins and in the body there are none. Could you explain it?

DR. LITWIN: I used these findings as indirect evidence for regulatory gene defects. There are few data on the nature of the defect. Spleen cells from certain strains of inbred mice exhibit a dissociation of *in vivo* and *in vitro* antibody response to sheep red cells with larger numbers of plaque forming cells detected *in vitro*. Dr. R.E. Click demonstrated that the *in vivo-in vitro* relationship was under genetic control for 19s antibody.

KURT HIRSCHHORN: A word about the frequencies of the X-linked and autosomal forms of combined immunodeficiency disease and the conclusion derived from the sex ratio of the patients.

If we have two forms of inheritance, X-linked and autosomal recessive and we call the frequencies of the disease X_1 for the X-linked and X_2 for the autosomal recessive form, then we know that the gene frequency for the X-linked condition is equal to the frequency of the disease and if we call q_1 the X-linked gene frequency, this equals S_1. On the other hand, in autosomal recessive diseases — with an equal frequency, in this case X_2, the frequency of these homozygous affected individuals is, in fact, q_2^2 because the distribution of normal heterozygotes and affected homozygotes is as $p^2:2pq:q^2$ with p and q being the gene frequencies for the normal and mutated genes. Therefore, in a situation where $X_1 = X_2$, you can also say that $q_1 = q_2^2$. For example, if the frequency of the X-linked condition is one in 10,000, so that $X_1 = X_2 = 0.0001$, then the frequency of the mutated gene for the X-linked (namely, q_1) also equals 1/10,000. The frequency of the autosomal recessive gene q_2 equals the square of this or one in one hundred (0.01). In other words, if the conclusion is correct, that the sex ratio of 3 to 1 implies an equal frequency of autosomal recessive and X-linked types, and if we make the oversimplified assumption that the autosomal recessives are all due to one gene, then the frequency of the mutated gene for the autosomal recessive is one hundred times as frequent (using the numerical example given above) as is that for the X-linked gene.

BYUNG PARK (Harbor General Hospital, Torrance, California): Did you imply that one of your patients with agammaglobulinemia has a serum factor which inhibits the secretion of immunoglobulin with B lymphocytes?

DR. ROSEN: More than one. We have several common variable patients whose serum will inhabit normal B cells secreting immunoglobulins *in vitro*.

NIEVES M. ZALDIVAR (Mt. Sinai Hospital, New York, New York): If you have to hypothesize that immunoglobulins are produced *in vitro* by this patient's cells in the short term and long term cell lines but not *in vivo*, do you think that there might be a repressor *in vivo* or that you are giving these cells factors that are lacking *in vivo* when you give them media *in vitro?*

DR. LITWIN: I can only speak about long term cultured lymphoid cells. I favor a repressor mechanism along the lines of the case mentioned by Dr. Rosen rather than the absence of a required factor. Also, the nature of the immune response is such that any defect in proliferation could interfere with the immune response. In fact, there is really an extraordinary number of biological levels we could examine to explain the above phenomenon.

DR. MEUWISSEN: Your patient could be lacking an enzyme that is supplied *in vitro.*

DR. LITWIN: This is possible. Since most current data on the characteristics of long term cultured human lymphoid cells indicate that they are related to lymphocytes, you are suggesting that the missing enzyme is synthesized by cultured cells but not lymphocytes *in vivo* in affected persons.

DR. MEUWISSEN: I think there is a possibility that you might supply something in your culture medium.

RICHARD ALBERTINI (University of Vermont, College of Medicine, Burlington, Vermont): You're really talking about the possible role of cell kinetics. You contrive the situation *in vitro* by controlling the numbers of the cells involved, so perhaps you're dealing with a quantitative and not qualitative difference.

DR. LITWIN: When you study *in vitro* cultured human lymphoid lines derived from persons who are normal and persons who are diseased and try to compare them, you have the problem of the tremendous range of immuno-globulin production both in variety and amount. We are having to struggle to establish reasonable base lines as to what a cultured lymphoid cell, selected under esoteric culture conditions, produces. So, I think it is difficult at this point to apply kinetics *in vitro* because of the difficulty with the controls.

DR. ALBERTINI: I don't suggest applying kinetics. A difference in kinetics could explain the production *in vitro* versus the absence or low production *in vivo*. There could be a quite simple explanation rather than a repressor.

DR. LITWIN: I agree.

SECTION II

HUMAN PURINE METABOLISM*

Irving H. Fox

Purines are intricately interwoven into human intermediary metabolism as substrates, cofactors and regulatory molecules. Specialized functions of these compounds include a role in cell energy transport, nucleic acid synthesis, vasodilation, neurotransmission and platelet aggregation.

Purine metabolism refers to a complicated series of enzyme reactions which synthesize, catabolize and transform purine compounds. These pathways have attracted great interest in clinical medicine as a result of their relevance to a number of disease states. Hyperuricemia and gout, which afflict as many as 1 to 2% of the North American population, are most likely related to disorders of purine metabolism in a large proportion of cases. The description and elucidation of inborn errors of purine metabolism have added a wealth of information concerning the function and regulation of these pathways in man. Many drugs used for cancer chemotherapy or immunosuppression, such as azathioprine, 6-mercaptopurine and methotrexate, inhibit one or more reactions of purine biosynthesis.

Purine biochemical pathways may be subdivided into biosynthesis *de novo* nucleotide interconversions, salvage pathways and catabolic reactions. In-born errors of metabolism have been described in most of these subdivisions (Table 1).

Purine Biosynthesis De Novo (Fig. 1)

Purine biosynthesis *de novo* is a pathway leading to the synthesis of inosine-5'-monophosphate (IMP) from nonpurine precursors. In the first reaction, phosphoribosylpyrophosphate (PRPP) is synthesized from ATP and ribose-5-phosphate. The next reaction, the PRPP amidotransferase, is the first enzymatic step committed specifically to purine synthesis. In this reaction, the pyrophosphate group of PRPP is displaced by the amide group of

*This review was made possible by grants from the Medical Research Council of Canada (MA4758), the Canadian Arthritis and Rheumatism Society and the Ontario Heart Foundation.

TABLE 1

INBORN ERRORS OF HUMAN PURINE METABOLISM

COMPONENTS OF PURINE METABOLISM	INBORN ERRORS
1. PURINE BIOSYNTHESIS DE NOVO	a) PRPP SYNTHETASE MUTANT b) GLUTAMINE PRPP AMIDOTRANSFERASE MUTANT
2. NUCLEOTIDE INTERCONVERSIONS	NONE KNOWN
3. SALVAGE PATHWAYS	a) LESCH - NYHAN SYNDROME b) PARTIAL HG - PRT DEFICIENCY c) PARTIAL A - PRT DEFICIENCY
4. PURINE CATABOLISM	a) ADENOSINE DEAMINASE DEFICIENCY IN CID b) XANTHINURIA c) ELEVATED XANTHINE OXIDASE

REGULATION OF HUMAN PURINE METABOLISM
(abbreviated summary)

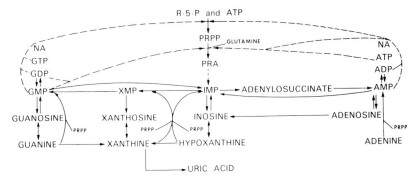

Fig. 1. Regulation of human purine metabolism. There are four major components of this pathway. (A) Purine biosynthesis *de novo* are those reactions which go from R-5-P and ATP to IMP. The PRPP synthetase enzyme catalyzes the reaction between ATP and R-5-P and the PRPP amidotransferase enzyme catalyzes the reaction between PRPP and glutamine. These 2 reactions are regulated in part by end product inhibitors (indicated by dotted lines). (B) Purine interconversions are those pathways by which IMP is converted to AMP and GMP and back again. (C) The purine salvage pathways include adenine phosphoribosyltransferase which catalyzes the conversion of adenine to AMP in the presence of PRPP and hypoxanthine-guanine phosphoribosyltransferase which catalyzes the conversion of hypoxanthine, guanine or xanthine in the presence of PRPP to IMP, GMP or XMP respectively. (D) Purine ribonucleotide catabolic pathways which lead from nucleotides to uric acid are explained in Figure 2. R-5-P, ribose-5-phosphate; ATP, adenosine triphosphate; ADP, adenosine diphosphate; AMP, adenosine monophosphate; PRPP, phosphoribosylpyrophosphate; PRA, phosphoribosylamine; IMP, inosine monophosphate; XMP, xanthosine monophosphate; GMP, guanosine monophosphate; GDP, guanosine diphosphate; GTP, guanosine triphosphate; NA, nucleic acid. (Figure 1 is reprinted with permission of Grune & Stratton, Inc., from I.H. Fox and W.N. Kelley, *Metabolism 21,* 713, 1972.)

47

glutamine to form phosphoribosylamine (PRA).

The regulation of these two reactions by intracellular PRPP and purine nucleotides has a major role controlling the whole reaction sequence of purine biosynthesis *de novo*. Intracellular PRPP is an essential substrate for several phosphoribosyltransferase reactions including the PRPP amidotransferase, the two purine salvage pathways, pyrimidine biosynthesis *de novo* and pyridine metabolism.[1] Under normal conditions, the intracellular concentration of PRPP (to 20 μM) in human tissues is substantially lower than the Km for the PRPP amidotransferase (500 = M).[2] As a result, depletion of PRPP *in vivo* and *in vitro* diminishes the rate of purine biosynthesis *de novo,* while elevation of PRPP causes increased activity of this pathway. This relationship provides an explanation for the existence of certain inborn errors of purine metabolism characterized by both elevated intracellular PRPP concentration and increased activity of purine biosynthesis *de novo*. In the Lesch-Nyhan syndrome, which is related to a deficiency of hypoxanthine-guanine phosphoribosyltransferase, PRPP levels are 10 times the normal concentration as a result of decreased utilization of this compound.[1,3,4] Two recently described PRPP synthetase variants with gout and overproduction of uric acid[5,6] are characterized by increased synthesis of PRPP with erythrocyte PRPP concentrations 2 to 3 times the normal concentration. This relationship also provides an explanation for the effects of specific drugs which reduce intracellular PRPP concentrations and inhibit purine biosynthesis *de novo*.[1] These compounds, substrates for phosphoribosyltransferase enzymes, include allopurinal, nicotinic acid, orotic acid, adenine and 2,6-diaminopurine.

Feedback inhibition of the first 2 steps of purine biosynthesis by nucleotides provides another potent mechanism of control. PRPP synthetase is regulated by heterogeneous nucleotide pool inhibition where most nucleotides bind at the same inhibitory site on the enzyme as well as by the cell energy charge and 2,3-diphosphoglycerate concentrations.[7] In contrast, PRPP amidotransferase is inhibited synergistically by two types of purine nucleotides. A combination of 6-amino (ex AMP) and 6-hydroxyl (ex GMP) nucleotides produced a substantially greater inhibition than was observed with equal concentrations of either nucleotide alone. Nucleotide end products also interact with PRPP to control the activity of the PRPP amidotransferase enzyme by shifting the substrate velocity curve from a hyperbolic to a sigmoidal function.[2] As a result of this effect, these nucleotides are strong inhibitors at the usual intracellular PRPP concentration.

The known inborn errors of the *de novo* pathway in man accelerate this reaction sequence by altering the regulatory mechanisms described above. This leads to the overproduction of uric acid, hyperuricemia and possibly gouty arthritis. Two types of PRPP synthetase mutants have been found. In one type, there was an increase in the Vmax of the enzyme,[6] while in the other, PRPP synthetase was insensitive to feedback inhibition by end products.[5] The net effect is increased intracellular PRPP concentration which stimulates PRPP amidotransferase activity. In another inborn error, the PRPP amidotransferase was insensitive to feedback inhibition from end products.[8] This represents a loss of an essential regulatory mechanism.

Nucleotide Interconversions (Fig. 1)

The purine nucleotide interconversion pathways are a complexly regulated series of reactions which allow the conversion of IMP to GMP and AMP and reconversion of these compounds to IMP. Although there are no human inborn errors of this pathway described, inosinic acid dehydrogenase, responsible for the conversion of IMP to XMP, is elevated in erythrocytes from the Lesch-Nyhan syndrome.[9]

Salvage Pathways (Fig. 1)

The purine salvage pathways include adenine phosphoribosyltransferase, which catalyzes the conversion of adenine and PRPP to AMP, and hypoxanthine-guanine phosphoribosyltransferase which catalyzes the conversion of PRPP and hypoxanthine, guanine or xanthine to IMP, GMP or XMP respectively. These pathways function to reutilize purine bases from nucleic acid catabolism and dietary purines for the synthesis of their respective ribonucleotide derivatives. Certain tissues, such as the brain and mature erythrocyte, utilize these pathways for the synthesis of purine nucleotides since purine biosynthesis *de novo* is absent. These pathways represent an economical means of forming nucleotides from an energy point of view since they utilize only 1 ATP as compared to 5 ATP's for the *de novo* pathway. The important role of the HG-PRT is emphasized by the 20 fold increase in purine biosynthesis in patients who have an almost complete deficiency of this enzyme.[10,11] The salvage pathways are regulated by their end products, including adenine and guanine nucleotides. Inborn errors of the reutilization include: (a) the Lesch-Nyhan syndrome, a complete deficiency of hypoxanthine-guanine phosphoribosyltransferase; (b) partial deficiency of hypoxanthine-guanine phosphoribosyltransferase, a syndrome described by Kelley *et al.,* comprising hyperuricemia, gout, overproduction of uric acid and, in some patients, neurological abnormalities;[12] and (c) partial deficiency of adenine phosphoribosyltransferase, an abnormality described only in erythrocytes and not definitely associated with a specific disorder of purine metabolism.[13,14]

Purine Ribonucleotide Catabolism (Fig. 2)

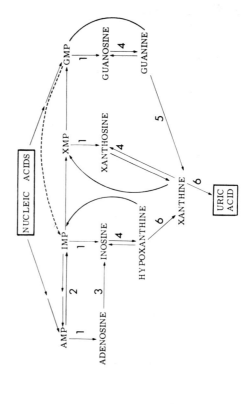

Fig. 2. Purine catabolism. Three major pathways lead from nucleotides to uric acid: (A) inosine is converted to hypoxanthine, xanthine and uric acid; (B) xanthosine is converted to xanthine and uric acid; (C) guanosine is converted to guanine, xanthine and uric acid. (1) dephosphorylation reaction by 5'-nucleotidase or non-specific phosphatase; (2) AMP deaminase; (3) adenosine deaminase; (4) purine nucleoside phosphorylase; (5) guanase; (6) xanthine oxidase.

50

The intracellular nucleotide pool is a dynamic balance between utilization and synthesis. Purine ribonucleotides are synthesized by purine biosynthesis *de novo*, the purine salvage pathways and the breakdown of nucleic acids. Nucleic acid synthesis, energy metabolism, cofactor synthesis and degradation to uric acid consume the nucleotide pool. Purine ribonucleotide catabolism refers to the sequence of reactions by which nucleotides are converted to uric acid, the end product of human purine metabolism.

Adenosine deaminase, deficient in combined immunodeficiency disease, catalyzes a reaction in the ribonucleotide catabolic pathway. We will consider these pathways in detail.

Three major pathways lead from nucleotides to uric acid: (a) AMP and IMP are converted to inosine, hypoxanthine, xanthine and then uric acid; (b) XMP is converted to xanthosine, xanthine and uric acid; (c) GMP is converted to guanosine, guanine, xanthine and uric acid. Ribonucleotide catabolism proceeds initially through a dephosphorylation step to form the ribonucleoside derivatives. 5′-phosphomono-esterase and non-specific alkaline and acid phosphatases hydrolyze AMP, IMP, XMP and GMP to adenosine, inosine, xanthosine and guanosine respectively. These enzymes are localized mainly to microsomal cell fractions with the highest specific activities in the plasma membrane. They are regulated by the nucleotide pool and inorganic phosphate concentration.[15–17] Allosteric inhibitory kinetics have been demonstrated for nucleoside triphosphates with sheep brain 5′-nucleotidase.[17] The purine nucleosides, inosine, xanthosine and guanosine, are converted to purine bases and ribose-1-phosphate by a nucleoside phosphorylase enzyme. Little or no adenosine is degraded to adenine by this reaction. In mammalian tissues, adenine nucleotide and nucleoside catabolism proceeds through IMP and inosine. This pathway appears to be important for nucleotide degradation since adenine nucleotides comprise a substantial proportion of the nucleotide pool with ATP forming approximately 60% of the total nucleoside triphosphates. The conversion of AMP to IMP has been studied in detail in calf brain and rabbit muscle where ATP and GTP have been found to have a complex regulatory role.[18–22] Adenosine is deaminated to inosine by adenosine deaminase in a number of mammalian tissues. Erythrocyte adenosine is sensitive to inhibition by purine ribonucleosides (Ki 8μM)[23] and related analogs, although little else is known of its regulation.

The catabolic pathway which has generated hypoxanthine from AMP and IMP, xanthine from XMP and guanine from GMP, ultimately forms uric acid. Guanine is deaminated to xanthine by guanase which has the highest activity in mammalian brain and hepatic tissues. The enzyme appears to be regulated by a protein inhibitor and GTP.[24,25] Hypoxanthine and xanthine are converted to uric acid by xanthine oxidase located primarily in the liver and jejunum of mammals. The regulation of xanthine oxidase activity by enzyme induction has been observed experimentally.[26]

Evidence from *in vitro* studies suggests that the intracellular concentration of ATP has an essential role in the regulation of the ribonucleotide catabolic pathway. Initial studies in respiring Krebs ascites tumor cells, using 2-deoxyglucose, revealed that the phosphorylation of this compound induced the loss of high energy phosphate in the form of ATP.[27] There was a concomitant rise in cellular AMP levels, a rise and later fall in IMP concentration until it became the predominant purine compound present. In Ehrlich ascites tumor cells under aerobic conditions, glucose caused a transient depletion of the adenine nucleotide pool which was initially similar to the 2-deoxyglucose effect.[28] The same events have been precipitated by glucose and 2-deoxyglucose during the study of the degradation steps of the purine nucleotide cycle of rabbit muscle extract.[29] These observations indicated that reactions which degrade AMP were accelerated by the sudden decrease in ATD concentration.

The pathways of ribonucleotide catabolism can be activated *in vivo* in man and other mammalian species. Perheentupa *et al.* initially observed the phenomenon of hyperuricemia following the intravenous infusion of fructose.[30] Subsequent observations demonstrated that within 30 minutes of fructose infusion, there was a marked total adenine nucleotide depletion with the most pronounced effect on intracellular ATP concentration in both rat liver[31] and human liver.[32] In perfused rat liver, fructose administration was followed by the accumulation of fructose-1-phosphate and alteration of intracellular intermediates[33] similar to the *in vitro* metabolic changes induced by 2-deoxyglucose.

More recent experiments by Fox and Kelley[34] have confirmed that pareneral fructose elevated the serum urate concentration. Their data supports the hypothesis that this hyperuricemia is related to stimulation of ribonucleotide catabolism rather than a direct stimulation of purine biosynthesis *de novo* or diminution of the renal clearance of uric acid. In this study, profound changes in purine metabolism were reflected in the serum by a mean 35% rise in serum uric acid within 30 minutes and in the urine by a mean 300% elevation of oxypurines, mainly hypoxanthine, a 144% increase in uric acid and the new appearance of inosine within 60 minutes of fructose infusion (Fig. 3). These observations demonstrate striking and abrupt changes in uric acid synthesis when the normal regulatory mechanisms inhibiting ribonucleotide catabolism are suddenly disrupted *in vivo*. The intracellular decrease of ATP and inorganic phosphate, resulting from the accumulation of a phosphorylated intermediate which is only slowly metabolized, releases the physiological inhibition of 5′-nucleotidase and AMP and adenosine deaminase. This results

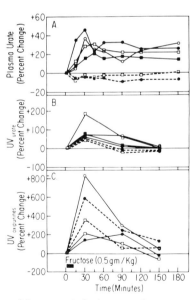

Fig. 3. Effect of fructose infusion on plasma urate and urinary excretion of uric acid and oxypurines. Results are expressed as percent change of control. Solid lines indicate no allopurinol, broken lines indicate pretreatment with allopurinol. (From Fox and Kelley, 1972.)

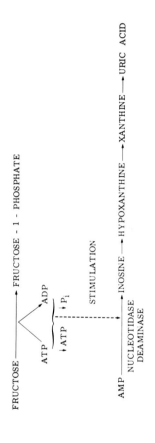

Fig. 4. Mechanisms of fructose induced hyperuricemia. The phosphorylation of fructose to fructose-1-phosphate causes a decrease in intracellular ATP and inorganic phosphate (Pi). This stimulates AMP breakdown to inosine by removing the usual inhibitory effect of these two compounds. Increased synthesis of hypoxanthine, xanthine and uric acid results.

in the stimulation of ribonucleotide catabolism (Fig. 4).

A number of inborn errors of ribonucleotide catabolism have now been described. Adenosine deaminase deficiency is being discussed in detail at this meeting. Xanthinuria, an autosomal recessively inherited deficiency of xanthine oxidase, is characterized by hypouricemia, diminished urinary urate excretion, elevated urinary oxypurine excretion and xanthinecalculi.[35] Primary gout has been described with elevated liver xanthine oxidase.[36] Since xanthine oxidase is inducible, it is unclear whether this enzyme increase is the primary abnormality or secondary to the presence of gout.

To summarize, human purine metabolism refers to a complex series of biochemical reactions by which purine compounds are synthesized, interconverted, reutilized and catabolized. The recent "purine revolution" has evolved in part with the discovery of inherited diseases of this pathway and with the development of clinically useful drugs that modify purine metabolism. The description of the adenosine deaminase deficiency in association with immunological abnormalities reveals new and exciting areas for exploration in both human purine metabolism and immunology.

REFERENCES

1.   I.H. Fox and W.N. Kelley, *Ann. Int. Med. 74,* 424, 1971.

2.   E.W. Holmes, J.A. McDonald, J.M. McCord, J.B. Wyngaarden and W.N. Kelley, *J. Biol. Chem. 248,* 144, 1973.

3.   F.M. Rosenbloom, J.F. Henderson, I.C. Caldwell *et al., J. Biol. Chem. 243,* 1166, 1968.

4.   M.L. Greene and J.E. Seegmiller, *Arth. Rheum. 12,* 666, 1969.

5.   O. Sperling, P. Boer, S. Persky-Brosh, E. Kanarek and A. DeVries, *Rev. Europ. Etudes Clin. et Biol. 17,* 703, 1972.

6.   M.A. Becker, L.J. Meyer, A.W. Wood and J.E. Seegmiller, *Science 179,* 1123, 1973.

7.   I.H. Fox and W.N. Kelley, *J. Biol. Chem. 247,* 2126, 1972.

8.   J.F. Henderson, F.M. Rosenbloom, W.N. Kelley *et al., J. Clin. Invest. 47,* 1511, 1968.

9.   D.M. Pehlke, J.A. McDonald, E.W. Holmes *et al., J. Clin. Invest. 51,* 1398, 1972.

10.   M. Lesch, W.L. Nyhan, *Am. J. Med. 36,* 561, 1964.

11.   W.N. Kelley, F.M. Rosenbloom, J.F. Henderson *et al., Proc. Nat. Acad. Sci. USA 57,* 1735, 1967.

12.   W.N. Kelley, M.L. Greene, F.M. Rosenbloom *et al., Ann. Int. Med. 70,* 155, 1969.

13.   W.N. Kelley, R.I. Levy, F.M. Rosenbloom *et al., J. Clin. Invest. 47,* 2281, 1969.

14.   I.H. Fox, J.L. Meade and W.N. Kelley, *Am. J. Med.* (In press)

15.   C.S. Song and D. Bodansky, *J. Biol. Chem. 242,* 694, 1967.

16.   C.C. Widnell and J.C. Unkeless, *Proc. Nat. Acad. Sci. 61,* 694, 1967.

17.   P.L. Ipata, *Biochem. 7, 507,* 1968.

18.   K.L. Smiley, Jr., A.J. Berry and C.H. Suelter, *J. Biol. Chem. 242,* 2502, 1967.

19.   K.L. Smiley, Jr. and C.H. Suelter, *J. Biol. Chem. 242,* 1980, 1967.

20.   B. Setlow, R. Barger and J.M. Lowenstein, *J. Biol. Chem. 241,* 1244, 1966.

21.   B. Setlow and J.M. Lowenstein, *J. Biol. Chem. 242,* 607, 1967.

22.   B. Setlow and J.M. Lowenstein, *J. Biol. Chem. 243,* 3409, 1968.

23.   W.R.A. Osbome and N. Spencer, *Biochem. J. 133,* 117, 1973.

24.   S. Kumar, *Arch. Biochem. Biophys. 130,* 693, 1969.

25.   V. Josan and P.S. Kirschman, *Biochem. Biophys. Res. Commun. 32,* 229, 1968.

26.   P.B. Rowe and J.B. Wyngaarden, *J. Biol. Chem. 241,* 5571, 1966.

27.   R.B. McComb and W.D. Yushok, *Can. Res. 24,* 198, 1964.

28.   K. Overgaard-Hansen, *Biochim. Biophys. Acta 104,* 330, 1965.

29.   J.M. Lowenstein, *Physiol. Rev. 52,* 382, 1972.

30.   J. Perheentupa and K. Raivio, *Lancet II,* 528, 1967.

31. K.O. Raivio, M.P. Kekomaki and P.J. Maenpaa, *Pharmacol. 18,* 2615, 1968.

32. L. Bode, H. Schumacher, H. Goebell *et al., Horm. Metab. Res. 3,* 71, 1971.

33. H.F. Woods, L.V. Eggleston and H.A. Krebs, *Biochem. J. 119,* 501, 1970.

34. I.H. Fox and W.N. Kelley, *Metabolism 21,* 713, 1972.

35. J.B. Wyngaarden, *in* The Metabolic Basis of Inherited Disease, J.B. Stanbury, J.B. Wyngaarden and D.S. Fredrickson (Eds.), third edition, 992, 1972.

36. A. Carcassi, R. Marcolongo, Jr., E. Marinello *et al., Arth. Rheum. 12,* 17, 1969.

THE LESCH-NYHAN SYNDROME*

William L. Nyhan

The Lesch-Nyhan syndrome is a genetically determined disorder of purine metabolism first definitively described in 1964.[1] The responsible gene is on the X chromosome. The phenotype is an X-linked recessive characteristic. The molecular expression of the abnormal gene is in the defective activity of the enzyme hypoxanthine guanine phosphoribosyl transferase (HGPRT; E. C. 2. 4. 2. 8).[2] This disorder was the first disorder of purine metabolism in which there were far-reaching biological effects. Adenosine deaminase appears to be a second. These observations point up the importance of the metabolism of purines in the overall ecology of the body.

Clinical Picture

The cardinal clinical characteristics of the syndrome are mental retardation, spastic cerebral palsy, choreoathetosis and self-mutilative behavior.[3,4] These patients also have hyperuricemia and may develop gouty arthritis, tophi, urinary tract stone disease and nephropathy.

The Lesch-Nyhan syndrome occurs exclusively in males. Involved infants appear normal at birth and usually develop normally for the first six to eight months. Crystalluria, hematuria or renal tract stone disease may develop during these early months of life but in most patients the urological examination is negative.

The onset of cerebral manifestations is with athetosis. Infants who have been sitting and holding their heads up begin to lose these abilities. Initially, they may be hypotonic or hypertonic but deep tendon reflexes are increased. Later they are all markedly hypertonic. In the established disease, motor defect is of such severity that the patient can neither stand nor sit unassisted. None of our patients with the Lesch-Nyhan syndrome has walked. All of the patients described have been mentally retarded. The motor defect is of

*Aided by U.S. Public Health Service Research Grant No. GM 17702, from the National Institute of General Medical Sciences, National Institutes of Health, Bethesda, Maryland.

greater severity than the defect in intelligence but most of our patients have had IQs of 50 or less. None of the patients has been successfully toilet trained.

Involuntary movements of both choreic and athetoid type have been prominent. Choreoathetoid cerebral palsy may be the most consistent feature of the syndrome. Patients are particularly prone to sudden opisthotonus or extensor spasms of the trunk. Scissoring of the lower extremities is regularly observed. Deep tendon reflexes are increased. Some, but not all, patients have had positive Babinski signs. Many have had ankle clonus.

The speech is characterized by athetoid dysarthria. Athetoid dysphagia is another problem. These patients have so much difficulty swallowing that they are difficult to feed. They all vomit frequently. In a busy, crowded institution for the retarded, such patients may die of inanition. In addition, they aspirate frequently and pneumonia is common. Most of the patients are markedly underweight and many are quite short. The bone age may be retarded. Convulsions are not a regular feature of the syndrome but they have been observed in a number of patients.

Aggressive, self-mutilating behavior is probably the most striking aspect of the syndrome.[1,4] Self-mutilation may begin as early as the eruption of the teeth. It usually begins, at least, shortly thereafter. Most patients bite both their lips and fingers destructively. Every patient we have seen has bitten his lips destructively unless the primary teeth have been removed early. In most patients, the hallmark of the syndrome is loss of tissue about the lips. Partial amputations of the fingers are common.

Sensation is intact in children with the Lesch-Nyhan syndrome. They scream in pain when they bite themselves and it is clear that they really do not want to do what they are doing. They are really happy only when securely protected from themselves. Many of these children scream all night until their parents or guardians are taught how to restrain them securely in bed. As they grow older these children learn to call for help. The cry of the young child with the syndrome carries the same message. Mutilation in this syndrome is compulsive behavior. It does not take the form of biting alone. These children are generally self-destructive. They also will direct their aggressions against others. They do bite others. As they learn speech they become verbally aggressive.

The behavior of these patients is a striking and provocative element in the syndrome. To our knowledge, this is the first instance in which a stereotyped pattern of human behavior has been associated with a distinct biochemical abnormality. Understanding of the mechanism could contribute to an understanding of behavior and its biochemical basis.

Manifestations of Hyperuricemia

A number of clinical manifestations are related directly to the accumulation of uric acid in body fluids. Patients with this syndrome have hyperuricemia from the neonatal period. They are subject to all of the clinical manifestations of gout. Acute attacks of arthritis develop only after a number of years of hyperuricemia. Three of our older patients have had acute arthritis. An involved cousin of one patient was said to have died at 21 years and to have had repeated episodes of arthritis in his last year.

Hematuria and crystalluria are common. Very early there may be masses of orange crystalline material in the diapers. A number of patients have had urinary tract stones.[5,6] Infantile colic and recurrent abdominal pains in older children may relate to the presence of large amounts of insoluble material in the urine. Urinary tract infections have been common only in those with stones. Many of these patients develop a renal concentration defect with polyuria and polydipsia, as well as failure to concentrate the urine. These patients may have great difficulty satisfying their thirst in a large busy institution. Urate nephropathy may lead to renal failure and this has probably been the most common cause of early death.

Tophi also develop. We have seen tophi in three patients. One patient had a tophus on his ear that was as large as a golf ball. Another had tophi which broke down and drained solid white urate.

Metabolic Abnormalities

In most patients, the first evidence of metabolic abnormality is the elevated concentration of uric acid in the blood, usually in the range of 10 mg per 100 ml.

The excretion of uric acid in the urine is always elevated. Children with this syndrome excrete three to four times as much uric acid as do control children. They often excrete over 600 mg per day. Among adult patients with gout those who have excreted this much urate have been classified as hyperexcretors. Relative to the body weight, patients with the Lesch-Nyhan syndrome excrete from 40 to 60 mg per kg. In terms of the excretion of creatinine, these patients usually excrete 3 to 4 mg of uric acid per mg of creatinine, while control individuals excrete less than 1.

The metabolism of purines has been studied by determining the rate at which uric acid is synthesized from glycine. This has been done by administering isotopically labeled glycine. In our original studies, the tracer glycine was labeled with ^{14}C.[1,5,7] More recently, we have explored the utility of the nonradioactive isotope of carbon, ^{13}C, for these studies (Fig. 1). In either case, the uric acid must be isolated from the urine, purified and its isotope content determined. Isolated uric acid that is labeled with ^{14}C is added to a scintillation solution and counted directly. For ^{13}C-labeled uric acid, we have made tetramethyluric acid, using trimethylalanine

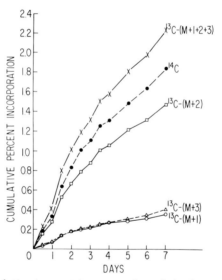

Fig. 1. Cumulative percent incorporation of the isotope of glycine-1-^{14}C and glycine-1, 2—[13]C into the urinary urate of a boy with Lesch-Nyhan syndrome. Each isotopically labeled compound was injected simultaneously. M + 1, M + 2 and M + 3 indicate the atom percent excess of the mass of uric acid plus one, two and three, atoms of [13]C. (Reprinted with permission from Sweetman *et al.,* Proc. Conf. Stable Isotopes in Chem., Biol. and Med., Argonne, Ill., May 1973, U.S. Atomic Energ. Comm., Natl. Techn. Inform. Serv.)[8]

hydroxide, purified it on a Sephadex G10 column and chromatographed it on a gas chromatographic inlet to a mass spectrometer with an alternating voltage accelerator.[8,9]

In patients, there is a rapid peak of specific activity in the first 24 hours. At the peak, it is easy to distinguish patients from controls. In studies of this sort in adults, it has not been possible to distinguish patients with gout from control individuals. Therefore, it has become conventional to express the data as the cumulative percent of the isotope of administered glycine that has been converted to uric acid. Adults with overproduction gout convert about twice as much glycine to uric acid as to controls. In children with the Lesch-Nyhan syndrome, about 2 percent of the glycine administered has regularly been recovered in uric acid.[1,5,7,8] This represents about 20 times the control value.[3] These are the highest rates of overproduction of purine reported.

Our studies using ^{13}C-labeled glycine have demonstrated that patients with Lesch-Nyhan syndrome have curves of specific activity as well as cumulative percent incorporation that are virtually identical to that obtained using ^{14}C-labeled glycine. Initially, we studied the simultaneous incorporation of both tracers in the same patient (Fig. 1). The high purity obtained by derivatization and the extra column purification leads to smoother curves for ^{13}C than for [14]C. Greater isotope enrichments obtainable with a non-radioactive tracer permit the assay of very small samples. We believe that this methodology will have many important applications in the *in vivo* study of man.

In the face of an overproduction of purine of this magnitude, there is an accumulation of compounds other than uric acid. These patients excrete xanthine in about the quantities found in normal urine. The amounts of hypo-xanthine are, however, markedly increased.[10,11] In most individuals, the molar ratio of hypoxanthine to xanthine is less than one. In these patients, the ratio is considerably greater than one and it may be as high as 8. When the patient is treated with allopurinol which inhibits xanthine oxidase, urate excretion decreases and other oxypurines become the major products of the overproduction. The hypoxanthine to xanthine ratio decreases with small doses of allopurinol but as the degree of the block is increased, more and more purine ends up as hypoxanthine. In controls treated with allopurinol, most of the oxypurine excreted is xanthine. These observations indicate that in normal individuals most urinary urate is formed from xanthine which does not come from hypoxanthine.

This is consistent with the occurrence of xanthinuria in patients with congenital absence of xanthine oxidase. These abnormalities are reflected in the central nervous system. Uric acid is not formed in the brain. These other oxypurines are the end-products of purine metabolism there. In the cerebro-spinal fluid,[12] xanthine concentrations are identical with those of controls. The concentrations of hypoxanthine in patients with the Lesch-Nyhan syndrome were some four times greater than in controls. Treatment with allopurinol increased the concentration of oxypurines in the cerebrospinal fluid of these patients even further.

The Molecular Defect — Deficient Activity of HGPRT

The primary site for the expression of the abnormal gene in the Lesch-Nyhan syndrome is the enzyme hypoxanthine guanine phosphoribosyl transferase (HGPRT) (Fig. 2). This enzyme converts the purine bases, hypoxanthine and guanine, to their respective nucleotides, inosinic and guanylic acids (IMP and GMP). The purine analogs, 6-mercaptopurine, 6-thioguanine and 8-azaguanine, require the presence of this enzyme and conversion to their respective nucleotides before they can become active chemotherapeutic or cytotoxic agents. Deficiency in the activity of HGPRT in the Lesch-Nyhan syndrome was first reported by Seegmiller, Rosenbloom and Kelley.[2] This important observation has been confirmed by a number of investigators.[13,14,15] The enzyme is normally present in all tissues of the body. In involved patients, activity is deficient in every tissue. It is most conveniently measured in the erythrocyte. Quantitative assay of the enzyme in the erythrocyte has regularly revealed no activity. The more precisely quantitative the determination, the more it is clear that the values obtained in patients cannot be distinguished from zero.

HGPRT may be studied by electrophoresis on polyacrylamide disc gel. The pattern for HGPRT is a reproducible one in which there is a broad area of activity with suggestions of resolution into four sub-bands.[16,17] Erythrocyte hemolysates from patients with the Lesch-Nyhan syndrome regularly yield an area of enzyme activity in this system.[17] Its mobility is faster than that of the normal enzyme but the activity is very low. These observations indicate that the mutation which produces this syndrome is in a structural gene and specifies a protein with an altered primary structure.

Genetics

The syndrome is found exclusively in males. Examination of several large kindreds in which there were a number of involved boys indicates that transmission is that of an X-linked recessive trait.[7]

Establishment of the deficiency of HGPRT activity permitted the molecular exploration of the genetics of the condition. In an X-linked recessive, the fathers should have normal activity of the enzyme and they do. The Lyon hypothesis specifies that the mothers, as heterozygotes, should be mosaics in

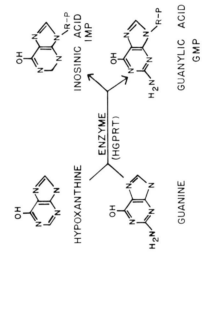

Fig. 2. The reaction catalyzed by hypoxanthine guanine phosphoribosyl transferase (HGPRT). This is the defect in the Lesch-Nyhan syndrome.

65

which there are two populations of cells, one completely normal and the other completely deficient. This has now been demonstrated by experiments in which fibroblasts in cell culture were cloned.[18,19]

However, assessment of the activity of HGPRT in erythrocytes or leukocytes of obligate heterozygotes for this condition, has always revealed normal HGPRT activity. Information on this subject has been obtained through the study of a key kindred in which two types of glucose-6-phosphate dehydrogenase (G6PD) were segregating as well as two types of HGPRT.[20] In this family, two sisters were heterozygous for HGPRT and for the G6PD types A and B. This was proven by cloning fibroblasts which were cultured from skin. However, repeated assay of their erythrocytes and leukocytes revealed only G6PD B as well as normal activity for HGPRT. These observations indicate a clonal origin of the hematopoietic system. The data could be explained by non-random inactivation of the X chromosome containing the information for G6PD and for HGPRT⁻. A more likely explanation is that there is random inactivation very early in fetal life but that it is followed by selection against the HGPRT⁻ cell.

Heterozygote Detection

The problem referred to in the last paragraph, which we have called hemizygous expression, has complicated the detection of heterozygotes in this condition. A molecular diagnosis of this type is essential for precise genetic counseling but it is clear that heterozygosity cannot be detected using the blood.

The presence of both cell types in cultures derived from their skin has permitted the use of fibroblasts in culture for diagnosis. Heterozygosity can, of course, be demonstrated by cloning.[18,19] However, the time, expense and attention involved preclude the use of cloning as a routine method for the diagnosis of the carrier of the gene. Pharmacological methods of cell selection[21,22] provide the cell culture method of choice for heterozygote detection. The principle of selection takes advantage of the unique properties of these cells. HGPRT is required for the activation of 6-mercaptopurine (6MP) and related analog inhibitors of purine metabolism. These include 6-thioguanine (6TG) and 8-azaguanine (AG). Normal cells containing HGPRT are killed by these compounds, while HGPRT⁻ cells are unaffected. Thus, in the mixed population of cells cultured from a heterozygote, this type of selective medium will permit the growth only of the HGPRT⁻ cells.

The assay of the enzyme in single hair follicles provides the most rapid, simple and least expensive method of heterozygote detection.[23-25] For routine use, it is probably the best method and promises to supplant methods requiring cell culture. It obviates the problem of selection *in vitro*. We have observed instances in which a single cell type grew out of a primary explant from the skin of a lady known to have two cell populations. It also obviates the problem of changes in enzyme content and activity during cultivation *in vitro*, which we have also observed. On the other hand, there are some technical problems. At least in our hands it is not always possible to obtain follicles. Cell culture methods may, therefore, be required if hair follicles cannot be obtained.

For validity, the hair follicle methods are dependent on the viability of cells and enzymes in each tiny follicle. Gartler and colleagues[23] have controlled this by splitting the extract obtained from each follicle and running both adenine phosphoribosyl transferase (APRT) and HGPRT. We do this electrophoretically and, therefore, can simultaneously assay both HGPRT and APRT on each single follicle. We believe it is well to assay 20 to 30 hairs for diagnosis.

Somatic Cell Genetics

Electrophoretic analysis indicates that the defect in the Lesch-Nyhan syndrome is the result of a structural gene mutation. This has been confirmed using antibody prepared in rabbits to normal erythrocyte HGPRT. Cross-reactive material has regularly been found in the cells of patients with the Lesch-Nyhan syndrome.[26, 27]

Heterogeneity is being increasingly recognized at the HGPRT locus. Ultimately, we believe that there will be a large number of different HGPRT proteins known and differences in the protein may be expected to lead to differences in the phenotype. It seems likely that one day a patient will be recognized in whom there is a defect in a regulator gene, although such a gene has not yet been defined.

Evidence for something like this has been obtained in studies of established HGPRT deficient lines in culture. In these lines, it is not too difficult to effect a cure *in vitro* by a process that might be called a form of genetic engineering.

Most HGPRT⁻ established cell lines have been developed by progressive selection for resistance in azaguanine or thioguanine from mouse, rat or hamster cells *in vitro*. They are usually tested by growth in azaguanine and failure to grow in hypoxanthine-aminopterin-thymidine (HAT) medium which kills any cell that does not have an active HGPRT.

Harris and colleagues[28,29] studied this system by fusing HGPRT⁻A9 cells of mouse origin with chick erythrocyte nuclei. Hybrid progeny cells in which no chick chromosomal material could be recognized grew in HAT, indicating the presence of HGPRT activity. From electrophoretic analysis, they concluded that the HGPRT was of chick origin.

We have undertaken similar studies using the mouse 1R cell. This cell is an HGPRT⁻ cell, which is convenient for study because it contains a marker chromosome. We fused these cells with chick embryo fibroblasts and obtained progeny cells which grew in HAT.[30] These progeny cells regularly contained the 1R marker chromosome. We subjected clones of these cells to our polyacrylamide gel electrophoretic method and found, without exception, that the HGPRT was that of the mouse, not the chick (Fig. 3). In similar experiments, we have fused HGPRT⁻FU5AH rat cells and HGPRT⁻Wg3 hamster cells with human WI 38 cells. In each instance, we have obtained clones in which the original rat HGPRT has been activated.

Several explanations are possible for these observations. We incline to the view that the deficiency of HGPRT in established lines is due to a mutation in a regulator gene and that fusion has supplied the regulator in the hybrids.

In any case, the experiment has interesting implications for possibilities of treatment in human genetic disease. The first condition may be that the defect is in a regulator rather than in a structural gene. However, it is possible that genetic material could be provided through hybridization that restored defective enzyme activity. If the restoration proved stable *in vitro,* there might be ways to provide it *in vivo,* such as through transplantation.

Treatment

There is currently no treatment which is of any benefit in the treatment or prevention of the central nervous system manifestations of the Lesch-Nyhan syndrome.

The renal complications of the hyperuricemia, as well as the arthritis and tophi, are effectively managed using allopurinol. The oral administration of allopurinol, in a dose of 200 to 400 mg a day, causes a reduction of plasma and urinary levels of uric acid and a concomitant increase in the oxypurines, hypoxanthine and xanthine.[10,11] In controls and in adults with gout and normal activity of HGPRT, the total excretion of oxypurines; i.e., the sum of uric acid, xanthine and hypoxanthine is less after treatment with allopurinol than under control conditions. In patients with this syndrome, this decrease in oxypurine excretion is not seen.[10] Probenecid and other uricosuric agents have been used in the management of this disease but we feel that uricosuric agents are contraindicated in patients with HGPRT deficiency. These individuals already process an enormous amount of renal urate. A uricosuric agent could lead to a renal shutdown and death. Alkali therapy with sodium citrate or sodium bicarbonate is effective in many patients who drink sufficient water to prevent crystalluria and stones and to maintain a normal level of urea nitrogen in the blood. However, this form of management is much more difficult than allopurinol therapy, particularly at times of intercurrent illness.

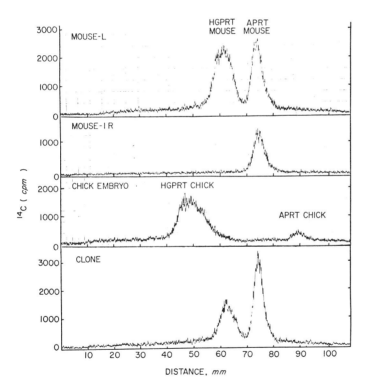

Fig. 3. Electrophoretic analysis of **HGPRT** and **APRT** isoenzymes in extracts of mouse L cells, mouse 1R cells, chick embryo fibroblasts and a clone derived by hybridizing 1R cells with chick embryo fibroblasts. (Reprinted with permission from *Proc. Nat. Acad. Sci. 70,* 1998, 1973.)[30]

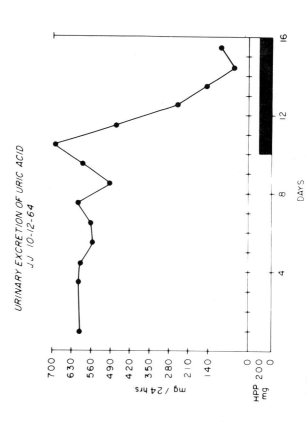

Fig. 4 Effect of allopurinal on the excretion of uric acid in the urine of a patient with the Lesch-Nyhan syndrome.

70

REFERENCES

1. M. Lesch and W.L. Nyhan, *Am. J. Med. 36,* 561, 1964.

2. J.E. Seegmiller, F.M. Rosenbloom and W.N. Kelley, *Science 155,* 1682, 1967.

3. W.L. Nyhan, *Fed. Proc. 27,* 1027, 1968.

4. W.L. Nyhan, *Arch. Int. Med. 130,* 186, 1972.

5. W.L. Nyhan, W.J. Oliver and M. Lesch, *J. Pediat. 67,* 257, 1965.

6. R.W. Howard and M.P. Walzak, *J. Urol. 98,* 639, 1968.

7. W.L. Nyhan, J. Pesek, L. Sweetman, D.G. Carpenter and C.H. Carter, *Pediat. Res. 1,* 5, 1967.

8. L. Sweetman, W.L. Nyhan, P.D. Klein and P.A. Szczepanik, *in* Proc. Conf. Stable Isotopes in Chem., Biol. and Med., Argonne, Ill., May, 1973, U.S. Atomic Energ. Comm., Natl. Techn. Infor. Serv. (in press).

9. P.D. Klein, J.R. Haumann and W.J. Eisler, *Anal. Chem. 44,* 490, 1972.

10. L. Sweetman and W.L. Nyhan, *Nature 215,* 859, 1967.

11. M.E. Balis, I.H. Krakoff, P.H. Berman and J. Dancis, *Science 156,* 1122, 1967.

12. L. Sweetman, *Fed. Proc. 27,* 1055, 1968.

13. B. Bakay, M.A. Telfer and W.L. Nyhan, *Biochem. Med. 3,* 230, 1969.

14. P.H. Berman, M.E. Balis and J. Dancis, *J. Lab. Clin. Med. 71,* 247, 1968.

15. L. Sweetman and W.L. Nyhan, *Arch. Int. Med. 130,* 214, 1972.

16. B. Bakay and W.L. Nyhan, *Biochem. Genet. 5,* 81, 1971.

17. B. Bakay and W.L. Nyhan, *Biochem. Genet. 6,* 139, 1972.

18. B.R. Migeon, V.M. Derkaloustian, W.L. Nyhan, W.J. Young and B. Childs, *Science 160,* 425, 1968.

19. J. Saltzman, R. DeMars and P. Benke, *Proc. Nat. Acad. Sci. 60,*

545, 1968.

20. W.L. Nyhan, B. Bakay, J.D. Connor, J.F. Marks and D.K. Keele, *Proc. Nat. Acad. Sci. 65,* 214, 1970.

21. J.S. Felix and R. DeMars, *J. Lab. Clin. Med. 77,* 596, 1971.

22. B.R. Migeon, *Biochem. Genet. 4,* 377, 1971.

23. S.M. Gartler, R.C. Scott, J.L. Goldstein and B. Campbell, *Science 172,* 572, 1971.

24. D.N. Silvers, R.P. Cox, M.E. Balis and J. Dancis, *New Eng. J. Med. 286,* 390, 1972.

25. U. Francke, B. Bakay and W.L. Nyhan, *J. Pediat. 82,* 472, 1973.

26. C.S. Rubin, J. Dancis, L.C. Yip, R.C. Niwinski and M.E. Balis, *Proc. Nat. Acad. Sci. 68,* 1461, 1973.

27. W.J. Arnold, J.C. Mead and W.N. Kelley, *J. Clin. Invest. 51,* 1805, 1972.

28. H. Harris and P.R. Cook, *J. Cell. Sci. 5,* 121, 1969.

29. A.G. Schwartz, P.R. Cook and H. Harris, *Nature New Biol. 230,* 5, 1971.

30. B. Bakay, C.M. Croce, H. Koprowski and W.L. Nyhan, *Proc. Nat. Acad. Sci. 70,* 1998, 1973.

IMPAIRMENT OF ADENOSINE DEAMINASE ACTIVITY IN COMBINED IMMUNOLOGICAL DEFICIENCY DISEASE*

Hilaire J. Meuwissen
Richard J. Pickering
Ellen C. Moore
Bernard Pollara

INTRODUCTION

Previously we have described a deficiency of the enzyme adenosine deaminase (ADA) in red blood cells (RBC) from 2 children with combined immunological deficiency disease (CID).[1-3] The combination of these rare defects in 2 patients suggested to us the possibility of a causal relationship between the 2 anomalies.

We have now investigated ADA activity in 8 patients with CID and have compared clinical and laboratory findings in patients with and without the enzyme deficiency. We have also measured ADA levels in red cells, serum and lymphocytes from parents of ADA deficient patients and from patients with other immunological deficiency disorders.

METHODS

Eight children were diagnosed as having CID on the basis of repeated infections early in life, impairment of lymphocyte function as measured by *in vivo* and *in vitro* methods (with or without lymphopenia), a paucity of lymphoid tissues and a variable deficiency of humoral immunity. Patients with other forms of immunodeficiency disease were seen at the Albany Medical Center Immunology Clinic. Normal adult male and female donors from the American Red Cross Blood Bank in Albany functioned as controls.

---

*Supported by PHS Grant HD 11717; National Institutes of Health Division of Research Resources, General Clinical Research Center, Grant 1-MO-RR00749; and the Canada Council.

73

ADA Deficiency

a. Red Blood Cells

Red blood cell ADA was measured in venous blood mixed with 15% acid citrate dextrose solution; blood was centrifuged three times at 200G and buffy coat removed after each sedimentation. One hundred μl of packed RBC's were added to 30 ml of 0.05 M phosphate buffer, pH 7.5, and sonicated for 3 minutes. Sonication was performed with a Branson M140 Sonicator (Heat Systems Ultrasonic, Inc., Plainview, New York) at 30 watts with the specimens immersed in ice. ADA activity in RBC sonicates was measured by the method of Hopkinson, using the increase in uric acid content as an index of ADA activity.[4] Red blood cell ADA was also assayed by thin layer chromatography and radioautography, using ^{14}C adenosine as precursor for the detection of inosine production.[5]

For histochemical demonstration of ADA in intact RBC, a modification of Fairbanks' method was used.[6] Venous blood was collected in 20% acid citrate dextrose solution, spun and the packed RBC's washed with saline. One hundred to 500 μl of packed RBC's were placed in freshly prepared sodium nitrate (Mallinckrodt, 0.18 M in saline) and incubated in a 37° C waterbath for 30 minutes. Twenty-five μl of washed packed erythrocytes were then added to tubes containing 0.4 ml adenosine (Sigma, 1 mg/ml), 0.2 ml Xanthine Oxidase (Boehringer, 10 μg/ml), 0.2 ml Phenazinium methosulfate (Baker, 0.5 mg/ml), 0.5 ml MTT Tetrazolium (Sigma, 2 mg/ml). All reagents were dissolved in 0.025 M phosphate buffer in normal saline, pH 7.0. Control groups were run without adenosine. After 20 minutes incubation in 37° C waterbath, the number of RBC's with formazan granules and the number of granules per RBC were read by microscopic examination.

b. Lymphocytes

Lymphocytes were purified on a Ficoll-Hypaque gradient, suspended at a concentration of 0.3×10^6/ml in a 0.05 M phosphate buffer and sonicated for 5 minutes. These lymphocyte preparations are contaminated by small numbers of macrophages, platelets and granulocytes.[7] ADA activity in the sonicate was measured by a modified Kalckar method[8] using 0.05 M phosphate buffer at pH 7.5 and 25 μgm adenosine per ml, or by the method of Karker.[10,11]

c. Sera and Tissues

ADA in serum, plasma or tissues was analyzed by the method of Goldberg,[9] or by measuring ammonia production, according to Karker's method.[10]

RESULTS

Three of the 8 patients with CID had complete absence of RBC-ADA activity as documented by spectrophotometric methods and by measurement of NH3 production (Table 1, Cases 1, 2 and 3, and Fig. 1). This group includes our patient T. Ha., who was described as the first case of ADA deficiency in an earlier report.[1] Histochemically, RBC's of ADA deficient patients contained 1 or 2 formazan granules per red cell in less than 1% of cells while more than 95% of RBC's from normal subjects contained several granules each (Fig. 2). In RBC's of T. Ha., no inosine production could be recorded by thin layer chromatography, indicating total absence of ADA activity by this method. Agarose and starch gel electrophoresis of red cell lysates showed a complete absence of all ADA bands in the 2 patients with CID and ADA deficiency who were examined (Table 1, Cases 1 and 3).

Lymphocytes from 1 patient with CID and red cell ADA deficiency (A. My.) showed no ADA activity when examined by Karker's methods,[10] while less than 5% of normal lymphocyte ADA activity was detected by the Kalckar method.[8] In 2 other patients (M. Re., T. Ha.) lymphocyte ADA was less than 5% of the normal level, and in one child (T. Ha.) tissue ADA was approximately 10% of normal. We were unable to study lymphocyte ADA by starch gel electrophoresis in any patient because a number of cells were not available. Sera from the 2 patients with red cell ADA deficiency who were examined failed to show any ADA activity (Table 1, Cases 1 and 3).

We have summarized clinical and laboratory data from our 8 patients with CID and added 3 other cases described in the literature[1,12] (Table 1). Five of the 11 patients have the enzyme deficiency. Four of the 6 patients with normal ADA levels were male and could have inherited CID in an X-linked manner: D. Ve. (Case 6) had a brother who died with documented CID;[13] M. Oc. (Case 9) had a maternal cousin who died with CID, while 3 other maternal cousins died in infancy from infection;[14,15] T. Be. (Case 8) had several maternal uncles and great uncles who died in infancy. By contrast, 4 of the 5 children with ADA deficiency were girls; the only boy in this group (M. Re.) had a sister with documented CID.[16] All patients had markedly depressed *in vitro* and *in vivo* T cell functions but the lymphopenia was more marked in the ADA deficient group. Furthermore, 2 of the 3 ADA deficient patients had unusual cupping and flaring of the costochondral junction of the ribs (patients A. My.[17,18] and M. Re.[18] – Table 1).

Five of the 6 parents of children with CID and ADA deficiency had red cell ADA levels which were more than 1 standard deviation below the mean on repeated testing (Fig. 1). Two parents with low RBC levels also had serum and lymphocyte ADA levels which were more than 1 standard deviation below the

TABLE 1

Clinical Findings in Patients with Combined Immunodeficiency Disease with and without ADA Deficiency

Patient	Sex	Lymphopenia	Antibodies	Associated Abnormalities
ADA Deficient				
(1) T.Ha.	F	Marked	Partial	Neutropenia S-IgA Deficiency
(2) M.Re.[a]	M	Marked	N.A.[b]	Bone Disease
(3) A.My.	F	Marked	Not detectable	Bone Disease Hypokalemia
(4) Detroit[c]	F	Variable	Partial	
(5) Denmark[d]	F	Marked?	None?	Hypoglycemia Hypokalemia
Normal ADA				
(6) D.Ve.[e,f]	M	Variable	Decreased	
(7) M.Pi.[a]	F	Mild	Not done	
(8) T.Be.[g]	M	Variable	Almost none	Hypoglycemia
(9) M.Oc.[h]	M	No	Partial	
(10) M.Vo.[h]	F	Mild	None	
(11) Denmark[d]	M	?	?	

a R.G.Keightley, A.R. Lawton, *Transpl. Rev. 16*, 15, 1973.
b Not applicable. Patient was transplanted in the first few weeks of life.
c F.Cohen: a sister died with thymus and thyroid hypoplasia(see Reference 1).
d J. Dissing (see Reference 12).
e M.A. South, Houston.
f In germ free environment from birth.
g R. Hong, Madison.
h A. Ammann, San Francisco.

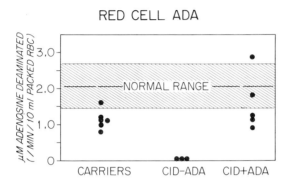

Fig. 1.   Red cell ADA was demonstrated by production of uric acid as described in the text.   Parents of children with CID and ADA deficiency are designated as "carriers".

CID-ADA: Patients with CID, with undetectable levels of ADA in red blood cells.

CID+ADA: Patients with CID and normal levels of ADA in red blood cells.

Normal range = Mean $\pm$ 1 S.D.

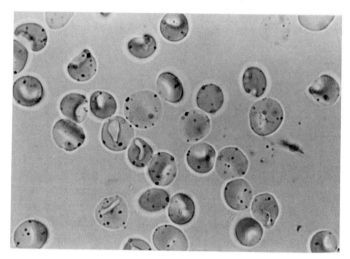

Fig. 2A. ADA in normal RBC's appear as formazan granules in virtually all cells.

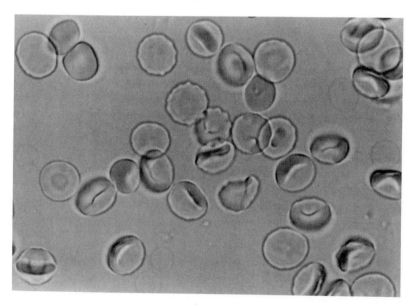

Fig. 2B. In patient with ADA deficiency few formazan granules are seen (see text).

mean on repeated testing (Fig. 1).

Patients with other forms of immunologic deficiency disease did not have evidence of red cell ADA deficiency. These included patients with hypogammaglobulinemia (variable form) (4 patients), transient hypogammaglobulinemia (4 patients), hypo-IgA (2 patients), Antibody-deficient syndrome (1 patient), Wiskott-Aldrich syndrome (2 patients), Ataxia telangiectasia (2 patients) and phagocytosis defect (2 patients). Three patients with drug-induced lymphopenia and hypogammaglobulinemia also had normal ADA levels in RBC's and serum.

DISCUSSION

The association between CID and ADA deficiency has been substantially confirmed by the present study. Five of 11 patients with evidence of CID are known to have had lack of ADA in their red cells. Two of these patients are known to lack serum ADA, while lymphocytes in 3 children contained less that 5% of normal ADA activity. The latter data were not available for the other 3 children with ADA deficiency. Absence of red cell ADA has not been seen so far in patients with other immune or non-immune disorders nor in any of several thousand normal subjects examined.[19,20] The recent finding of an apparently immunologically normal !Kung child with absent erythrocyte ADA is the single exception to these studies.[21] However, the levels of lymphocyte and serum ADA of this child are unknown. He may represent a unique human variant with normal lymphocyte and tissue ADA levels.[22]

Our data indicate that ADA deficiency is not a consequence of CID or of the lymphopenia seen in CID. Six of 11 patients with CID, several of whom had marked lymphopenia and hypogammaglobulinemia, had normal or near normal levels of ADA. Furthermore, patients with primary and secondary immunodeficiency involving B and T lymphocytes had normal ADA levels. Consequently, we have no evidence that immune deficiency by itself leads to ADA deficiency. It is possible, though highly unlikely, that ADA deficiency and CID both are caused by a single gene deletion and are, therefore, not causally related. Alternatively, ADA deficiency may have been produced by a mutation at the ADA locus and, in turn, may cause the immunological dysfunction seen in CID. We favor the latter hypothesis, primarily because the low residual ADA activity in tissues of T. Ha. mitigates against the gene deletion hypothesis.

Several studies indicate that ADA may plan an important role in lymphoid tissue function. Lymphoid organs, particularly spleen, contain a great amount of ADA in many mammalian species.[23–25] After antigenic stimulation of a regional lymph node, the level of ADA in efferent lymph rises together with the number of plasma cells and antibody concentration in the efferent lymph.[26] Serum ADA is elevated in malignant and non-malignant conditions, particularly those in which lymphoid cells proliferate rapidly.[27,28] Thus, ADA may play an as yet undefined role in proliferation or differentiation of lymphoid cells and possibly cartilage and bone. Other tissues may escape the effect of ADA deficiency because they proliferate less rapidly or because there is less need for diversity and continuous differentiation in these tissues.

The genetic control of ADA is not yet clear. A low molecular weight ADA is present in RBC's and many other body tissues, while a high molecular weight, slow-moving ADA appears to be specific for individual tissues, with the exception of the RBC's. The high molecular weight ADA is probably an aggregate of the low molecular weight ADA.[29] In the past, several ADA loci have been postulated to account for the phenotypic diversity of ADA,[25] but other investigations have now suggested the existence of a single ADA locus.[30,31] Patient No. 1 (T. Ha., Table 1) lacked ADA in her red blood cells and serum but had small amounts of ADA in all other body tissues examined.* These findings, however, are compatible with the single ADA gene hypothesis.

The studies reported here and those reported previously[1,12] suggest that parents of children with ADA deficiency are carriers of the enzyme abnormality. They have decreased levels of ADA in red cells, serum and lymphocytes. They appear clinically well, however, and extensive immunological evaluation of the mother of T. Ha. has revealed no abnormalities.**

If ADA deficiency is the cause of impaired immunological function in CID, new approaches to therapy of this disease may become available. As in many inborn errors of metabolism, an enzymatic block may lead to accumulation of a precursor substance or lack of a metabolite. In the patient's cells this may result in increased intracellular concentrations of adenosine, cyclic AMP[33] or other adenosine derivatives. On the other hand, lack of inosine may be deleterious for lymphocyte function.[34] If excessively high or low intracellular concentration of a metabolite crucial for lymphocyte function can be documented in purine metabolic pathways, it might be possible to devise corrective treatment of CID, using the principles that have been successfully used in phenylketonuria and other inborn errors of metabolism.[35]

---

*These tissues were previously analyzed by starch gel electrophoresis. By that technique no ADA was demonstrated in tissues (see Reference 31).
  **Personal observations.

ACKNOWLEDGEMENTS

These studies would not have been possible without the generous cooperation of Drs. A. Ammann, M.D. Cooper, R. Keightley, R. Hong and M.A. South, who permitted us to study their patients.

We thank Ms. Karen Parker, Dina Schreinemachers, Bernadette Cook and Mr. Andrew Stacy for technical assistance, Dr. A. Britton for providing us with blood samples, and Drs. I.H. Porter, E.B. Hook, F. Maley and R. Hirschhorn for helpful discussions.

REFERENCES

1. E. Giblett, J. Anderson, F. Cohen *et al., Lancet II,* 1067, 1972.

2. H.J. Meuwissen, E. Moore and B. Pollara, *Ped. Research 7,* 362/143, 1973.

3. H.J. Meuwissen, R.J. Pickering and B. Pollara, *in* Immunodeficiency Diseases in Man and Animal, D. Bergsma (Ed.), The National Foundation, 1974 (in press).

4. D.A. Hopkinson, P. Cook and H. Harris, *Ann. Hum. Genet. 32,* 361, 1969.

5. H.P. Raaen and F.E. Kraus, *J. Chromatography 35,* 531, 1968.

6. V.F. Fairbanks and L.T. Lampe, *Blood 31,* 589, 1968.

7. K. Parker, D. Schreinemachers and H.J. Meuwissen, *Transplantation 14,* 135, 1972.

8. H.M. Kalckar, *J. Biol. Chem. 167,* 461, 1947.

9. D.M. Goldberg, *Brit. Med. J. 1,* 353, 1965.

10. H. Karker, *Scand. J. Clin. Lab. Invest. 16,* 570, 1964.

11. E.M. Scholar, P.R. Brown, R.E. Parks, Jr. and P. Calabresi, *Blood 41,* 927, 1973.

12. J. Dissing and B. Knudsen, *Lancet II,* 1316, 1972.

13. M.A. Smith, J.R. Montgomery, R. Wilson *et al., Exp. Hematol. 22,* 71, 1972.

14. W.E. Hathaway, J.H. Githens, W.R. Blackburn *et al., N. Engl. J. Med.* *273*, 953, 1965.

15. A.J. Ammann, D.W. Wara, S. Salmon and H. Perkins, *N. Engl. J. Med.* *289*, 5, 1973.

16. R.G. Keightley, A.R. Lawton, L.Y. Wu *et al.*, This Symposium, p.

17. C.S. Kyong, B.St.J. Brown and R.J. Pickering, Personal Observation.

18. H.J. Meuwissen, B. Pollara and R.J. Pickering, *J. Pediat.* (in press).

19. J. Dissing and J.B. Knudsen, *Hum. Hered. 19*, 375, 1969.

20. J.C. Detter, G. Stamatoyannopoulos, E.R. Giblett and A.G. Motulsky,

21. T. Jenkins, *Lancet 2*, 736, 1973.

22. B. Pollara and H.J. Meuwissen, *Lancet 2*, 1324, 1973.

23. J.M. Barnes, *Brit. J. Exp. Path. 21*, 264, 1940.

24. T.G. Brady and C.O'Donovan, *Comp. Biochem. Physiol. 14*, 101, 1965.

25. Y. Edwards, D. Hopkinson and H. Harris, *Ann. Hum. Genet. (London) 35*, 207, 1971.

26. J.G. Hall, *Austral. J. Exp. Biol. 41*, 93, 1963.

27. M.K. Schwartz and O. Bodansky, *Proc. Soc. Exp. Biol. Med. 101*, 560, 1959.

28. L.H. Koehler and E. Benz, *Clin. Chem. 8*, 133, 1962.

29. H. Nishihara, S. Ishikawa, K. Shinkai and H. Akedo, *Biochim. Biophys. Acta 302*, 429, 1973.

30. N. Ressler, *Clin. Chim. Acta 24*, 247, 1969.

31. R. Hirschhorn, V. Levytska, H.J. Meuwissen and B. Pollara, *Nature, New Biol. 246*, 200, 1973.

32. E. Giblett, Workshop Report, This Symposium, p.

33. H. Green and T. Chan, *Science 182*, 836, 1973.

34. A. Glasky, This Symposium, p.

35. J.B. Stanbury, J.B. Wyngaarden and D.S. Fredrickson, The Metabolic Basis of Inherited Disease, McGraw-Hill, New York, 1972.

DISCUSSION

DR. MEUWISSEN: Dr. Nyhan, have you studied the immune responses in your patients with Lesch-Nyhan syndrome?

DR. NYHAN: We certainly have not studied this systematically but I do not think it is likely that they have a serious defect.

DR. ALBERTINI: Our laboratory had occasion to look at PHA responses in an entirely different context. It certainly wasn't studied well but we did not notice any difference between Lesch-Nyhan boys, heterozygous females or normals.

DR. MEUWISSEN: How many patients did you study?

DR. ALBERTINI: Six to eight.

DR. POLLARA: Dr. Fox, could adenosine be catabolized other than through the deaminase pathway?
In the face of increased intracellular levels of adenosine that one assumes may be found in patients with CID and ADA deficiency, would you expect accelerated conversion to AMP through the adenosine kinase system?

DR. FOX: As you have already mentioned, the two main pathways of adenosine metabolism are through adenosine deaminase and adenosine kinase. The question is whether there is a build up of intracellular adenosine and I am not sure what the concentration of intracellular adenosine is. I would suspect that a rise in intracellular adenosine would accelerate the adenosine kinase reaction. The effect of rising intracellular adenosine concentration on cyclic AMP metabolism must be considered since adenosine deaminase has a regulatory effect on adenyl cyclase activity. You need data on the change in intracellular nucleotides before you can really speculate any further.

ROBERT E. PARKS, JR. (Brown University, Providence, Rhode Island): In response to Dr. Pollara's question, I would like to point out that in addition to ADA there is another reaction pathway that can lead to the deamination of adenosine. This involves the enzyme $5'$-AMP deaminase. In other words, adenosine can react with ATP and adenosine kinase to form AMP which, in turn, can be deaminated by $5'$-AMP deaminase to form inosinic acid (IMP). The phosphate of IMP could then be hydrolyzed by $5'$-nucleotidases forming

85

inosine. The enzyme 5'-AMP deaminase appears to be an important regulator of nucleotide levels in cells and, in addition, may play a major role in tissues such as muscle in the deamination of amino acids. In fact, it appears that in muscle the adenylate cycle, which includes this enzyme, assumes the role played by glutamic dehydrogenase in tissues such as liver. A superb review of the adenylate cycle and the control of 5'-AMP deaminase was published by Lowenstein (*Physiol. Reviews 52,* 382, 1972). It will be interesting to examine cells from patients with ADA deficiency for the activity of 5'-AMP deaminase. I might expect that if the enzyme were not present and functioning in these cells, there would be no control on the uptake of adenosine into the nucleotide pools and extremely high concentrations of ATP would be found. The reason for suspecting this is that when we incubate erythrocytes with 2-fluoroadenosine, high concentrations of 2-fluoro-ATP are found in a relatively short time. In this case, 2-fluoroadenosine is resistant to deamination by ADA and we believe that the 2-fluoro-AMP formed in the adenosine kinase reaction is not a substrate for 5'-AMP deaminase.

There is a recent report from the University of Minnesota which suggests that you shouldn't be examining the effect of cAMP but rather of cGMP (J.W. Hadden, E.M. Hadden, M.K. Haddox and N.D. Goldberg, *Proc. Natl. Acad. Sci. 69,* 3024, 1972.

DR. LITWIN: There has been a great deal of interest in the role of both prostaglandins and cyclic AMP in the membrane surface during the immune response and I was wondering if we have any information on the levels of cyclic AMP or the build up of cyclic AMP which should occur during immune stimulation.

DR. MEUWISSEN: We don't. We have done a few experiments with lymphocytes of a carrier of ADA deficiency that did not give us specific answers.

DR. FREDMAN: Dr. Meuwissen, the last sentence in your paper was interesting. You said that ADA is the cause of combined immunological deficiency. Would you like to elaborate on this?

DR. MEUWISSEN: I feel it is most unlikely that ADA does not have something to do with lymphoid function.

DR. GERALD: Dr. Nyhan, do you find complete absence of the protein in your patients or do you find heterogeneity? I would expect wide variation — some deficient in the protein, others with a defective protein. In other words, are we dealing with a mutation of a regulator or structural gene?

DR. NYHAN: All of the evidence is that we are dealing with a mutation of a gene. A protein is present but its activity is extraordinarily low. With an electrophoretic method, we can show a little blip of activity. Whenever they've been looked at for a cross reacting immunoprotein, an enzyme has been present.

SECTION III

HUMAN CHROMOSOME MAPPING BY SOMATIC CELL HYBRIDIZATION*

P.S. Gerald

G.A. Bruns

The current remarkable progress in human chromosome mapping[1,2,3] results largely from the discovery by Weiss and Green that human-mouse somatic cell hybrids rapidly and progressively lose their human chromosomes.[4] In effect, a few human chromosomes become isolated in a "test tube" of mouse cytoplasm. Since the loss of human chromosomes is largely random, concordance of the presence or absence of two different human enzymes is preliminary evidence for the presence of their loci on the same chromosome.† Finally, correlation of residual human enzymes with the residual human chromosome present in the hybrids may be used to assign a syntenic group to a specific chromosome. (This will be referred to as assignment by concordance.)

The power of this new tool is remarkable. The present pace of progress is such that there is more data on gene assignment that is unpublished than is published. However, to avoid the uncertainty that necessarily attends quoting unpublished information, this presentation will deal only with published material as well as with studies currently underway in the author's laboratory.

The success of the hybrid cell technique depends on the ability of a cell from an established line to confer its growth characteristics on the hybrid cell. Since only a few hybrid cells are produced in any fusion experiment, removal of the excess established line parental cells is necessary in order to expose the few hybrid cells present. The use of selective systems which are lethal for the established cells but not for the hybrid is thus a central factor

---

*This work was supported in part by grants from the National Institutes of Health (No. HD04807, No. HD06285 and No. HD06276) and a grant from the Charles H. Hood Foundation.

†Loci which are present on the same chromosome are said to be syntenic;[5] two loci which are on different chromosomes are asyntenic. Linked loci are necessarily syntenic but not all syntenic loci are sufficiently near each other to exhibit linkage.

in somatic cell hybridization. The technique commonly employed at present utilizes an established cell line which is deficient in a given enzyme, the deficiency state having been produced by natural or induced mutation. The enzyme deficiency renders the cell inviable in a particular chemical environment. The enzyme deficiency thus not only allows for elimination of the established line parental cells but also forces survival of the hybrid cell to depend upon the enzyme produced by the genome of the non-deficient parent (Figure 1). Possession of the gene for this enzyme will usually mean possession of the chromosome which bears it.

In the hybrids used to map the human chromosomes, cells from an enzyme-deficient established line (most often mouse or Chinese hamster) are usually fused with diploid human fibroblasts or with leucocytes. When these hybrids are maintained in the selective system, only one particular human chromosome (that with the gene for the necessary enzyme) will be present in all cells. Those human enzymes which are uniformly present in such hybrids can with reasonable confidence be assigned to this chromosome. The chromosomes which have been most thoroughly analyzed by such "assignment by preferential survival" are listed in Table 1. It should be appreciated that assignment by preferential survival is more efficient but not different in principal from assignment by concordance.

The foregoing description of the use of somatic cell hybrids is over-simplified to the extent that a number of assumptions are made. Table 2 lists the more important of these assumptions. The first of these assumptions now seems to be well justified, although occasionally the mutant gene for the rodent enzyme deficiency may revert and once more produce functional rodent enzyme.[6,7] This phenomenon may have occurred twice or more in a series of 31 independently derived hybrids we have studied.

The second assumption, that the human chromosomes whose loci are not under selection will be randomly lost, has not yet been critically tested. The limited data presently available demonstrates that significant departures from randomness probably do occur. For example, chromosome 14 is present in about 80% of our hybrids while chromosome 1 is found only 40% of the time, as judged by the presence of enzymes assigned to these chromosomes. The observed departures from randomness are not sufficiently extreme to limit the usefulness of cell hybridization for gene assignment.

The most serious defect of present hybridization techniques is the tendency for the human chromosomes to undergo rearrangements in the hybrid cell. In our experience, one or more loci assigned to the human X are missing in approximately 10-20% of hybrid colonies maintained in medium selecting for that chromosome. Human chromosomes which are not involved in the selection process may also be broken, but with a lesser frequency. This

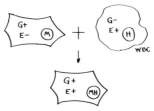

Fig. 1. Schematic representation of the fusion of a mouse cell and a human cell to form a human-mouse hybrid. A selective system is used to isolate the human-mouse hybrid. The mouse (M) established cell line has the ability to grow indefinitely in culture (G^+) but lacks an enzyme (E^-) necessary for survival when exposed to the selective system. The human (H) white blood cell (WBC) lacks the ability to grow (G^-) but possesses the enzyme (E^+) that permits survival in the selective system. The two factors (G^+ and E^+) required for growth are present only in the hybrid cell (MH) and the excess parental cell population is eliminated.

TABLE 1

Chromosome Assignment by Preferential Survival[2]

Chromosome X

    *Hypoxanthine-guanine phosphoribosyltransferase
    Glucose-6-phosphate dehydrogenase
    Phosphoglycerate kinase
    αGalactosidase

Chromosome 17

    *Thymidine kinase, soluble

Chromosome 16

    *Adenine phosphoribosyltransferase

---

    *Enzyme required for survival of the hybrid cell.

TABLE 2

Assumptions in Human Gene Assignment by Somatic Cell Hybridization

(1) Preferential survival of cells containing a specific human locus (and chromosome) occurs in medium selecting for enzyme determined by that locus.

(2) All other human chromosomes disappear randomly.

(3) Rearrangement of human chromosomes after fusion is infrequent.

(4) "Unexpected" regulatory effects only rarely alter the expression of human genes.

tendency to breakage necessitates that a considerable number of independently isolated hybrid colonies be examined before any conclusions can be drawn. The importance of this problem is illustrated by the fact that the several groups localizing genes to regions of the human X chromosome have not yet been able to reach general agreement.

The final major assumption is that regulatory effects will not confound the analysis. Most workers have implicitly assumed that enzymes active in both parental cells will have their expression in the hybrid cell determined solely by their respective structural genes. At present, it can only be said that there is no reason to question this assumption.

This analysis of the assumptions underlying somatic cell hybridization is not intended to sound a discouraging note but rather to emphasize that the power of the tool should not overwhelm our critical judgment and that the findings of cell hybridization must be confirmed by other techniques whenever possible. The history of assignment of loci to chromosome 1 (Table 3) provides an illustration of how results from various methodologies may be used to complement one another. Initially, the loci for 6-phosphogluconate dehydrogenase and the RH blood group were found to be linked by conventional recombinational analysis.[8] Next, the loci for the enzymes phosphoglucomutase (PGM$_1$), 6-phosphogluconate dehydrogenase and peptidase C were observed to be syntenic by hybrid cell studies.[9,10] Since this suggested that the Rh locus and the PGM$_1$ locus were on the same chromosome, linkage of the two loci was sought and successfully confirmed.[11,12] Finally, peptidase C was assigned to chromosome 1 by somatic cell hybridization.[13]

Most recently, an adenylate isozyme (AK$_2$)[14] and phosphopyruvate hydratase (PPH)[15] have been found by cell hybridization to be syntenic with one or more of the enzymes that have been assigned to chromosome 1. Dr. E. Giblett has independently obtained evidence for the assignment of PPH to chromosome 1 from a family in which an electrophoretic variant of PPH is linked with the Rh locus.[16] Table 3 summarizes the additive aspects of the information obtained from various sources.[13]

Table 4 lists the electrophoretically demonstrable enzymes whose loci have been assigned to human chromosomes. This table includes the abbreviations used in this paper, along with formally assigned numbers for the various enzymes[17] and the numbers available in McKusick's catalogue.[18] The chromosome to which each of these loci is assigned is given in Table 5. This information is taken from available publications[2,3] and from unpublished data in the author's laboratory. A recent workshop on human chromosome mapping brought to light conflicting data for certain of the loci in Table 5, so many of the assignments in this Table must be considered tentative.

TABLE 3

Genes Assigned to Chromosome 1

A.   By Somatic Cell Hybridization

     Peptidase C
     6-Phosphogluconate dehydrogenase
     Phosphoglucomutase − locus 1
     Adenylate kinase − locus 2
     Phosphopyruvate hydratase (enolase)

B.   By Linkage to Marker Chromosome 1

     Duffy blood group
     Pancreatic amylase

C.   By Linkage to Assigned Loci (A or B)

     Salivary amylase
     Congenital cataract
     Rhesus blood group

D.   By Linkage to Linked Loci (C)

     Auriculo-osteodysplasia
     Elliptocytosis

TABLE 4

Electrophoretically Demonstrable Enzymes Used In
Assignment Studies In Somatic Cell Hybrids

Enzyme	Abbrev.*	McKusick Cat. No.**	E.C. No. (17)
Acid phosphatase, lysosomal	AcP$_2$		
Adenosine deaminase	ADA	10270	3.5.4.4
Adenylate kinase (fibroblast)	AK$_2$		2.7.4.3
Adenine phosphoribosyltransferase	APRT	10260	2.4.2.7
Esterase-A$_4$	Es-A$_4$	13340	
αGalactosidase (Fabry's disease enzyme)	αGal	30150	3.2.1,22
Glucose-6-phosphate dehydrogenase	G6PD	30590	1.1.1.49
Glucosephosphate isomerase	GPI (PHI)	17240	5.3.1.9
Glutamate oxaloacetate transaminase, cytoplasmic	GOT$_1$	13825	2.6.1.1
Hypoxanthine-guanine phosphoribosyltransferase	HGPRT	30800	2.4.2.8
Indophenoloxidase-A, dimeric	IPO-D	14745	
Indophenoloxidase-B, tetrameric	IPO-T	14744	
Isocitrate dehydrogenase, cytoplasmic	IDH$_1$	14770	1.1.1.42
Lactate dehydrogenase-A	LDH-A	15000	1.1.1.27
Lactate dehydrogenase-B	LDH-B	15010	1.1.1.27
Malate dehydrogenase, cytoplasmic	MDH$_1$ (MOR)	15425	1.1.1.37
Malic enzyme, cytoplasmic	ME$_1$ (MOD)	15420	1.1.1.40
Mannose phosphate isomerase	MPI	15455	5.3.1.7
Nucleoside phosphorylase	NP	16405	2.4.2.1
Peptidase-A	Pep-A	16980	
Peptidase-B	Pep-B	16990	
Peptidase-C	Pep-C	17000	
Phosphoglucomutase$_1$	PGM$_1$	17190	2.7.5.1
Phosphoglucomutase$_3$	PGM$_3$	17210	2.7.5.1
6-Phosphogluconate dehydrogenase	PGD	17220	1.1.1.44
Phosphoglycerate kinase	PGK	31180	2.7.2.3
Phosphopyruvate hydratase	PPH		4.2.1.1
Pyruvate kinase (leucocytic form)	PK-III	17905	2.7.1.40
Thymidine kinase (cytoplasmic)	TK	18830	2.7.1.21

*The abbreviations used in this Table conform to the recommendations considered by a working party at a recent human chromosome mapping workshop held at Yale University (June, 1973).

**From V.A. McKusick, "Mendelian Inheritance in Man", 3rd Edition, The Johns Hopkins Press, Baltimore, 1971. Supplemented by personal communication.

TABLE 5

Assignment of Electrophoretically Demonstrable
Enzymes To Human Chromosomes By Somatic
Cell Hybridization

Chromosome No.	Enzyme*	Chromosome No.	Enzyme
1	PGD, PPH, PGM_1, Pep-C, AK_2	16	APRT
		17	TK
2	IDH_1, MDH_1		
		18	Pep-A
6	ME_1, IPO-T, PGM_3		
		19	GPI
7	MPI, PK-III		
		20	ADA
10	GOT_1		
		21	IPO-D
11	LDH-A, $Es-A_4$, AcP_2		
		X	αGal, PGK, HGPRT, G6PD
12	LDH-B, Pep-B		
14	NP		

*See Table 4 for abbreviations used.

In Table 5, the locus for adenosine deaminase (ADA), the enzyme of principal concern to this congress, is listed as assigned to chromosome 20. This assignment is only tentative at present since the original observation[2] has not yet been independently confirmed. Further, studies of this enzyme in hybrid cells have been complicated by the existence of isozymic species with differing molecular weights. Perhaps this conference will resolve the basic question of whether or not these several molecular species comprise a single gene entity.

The technique of somatic cell hybridization can also be used to localize assigned genes to a portion of a chromosome. This has been accomplished by using cells which contain a reciprocal translocation as in the human parental cell.[19] We have studied hybrids prepared from human cells containing a reciprocal translocation between an X and a chromosome 19 – t(Xq-; 19q+) – in which the translocated X is active. These cells have been fused with mouse and with Chinese hamster cells which lack HGPRT. In the selective system used, the translocation element containing the HGPRT locus, but not the other translocation element, is required for survival. In this way, hybrid cells containing only the distal portion of the long arm of the X have been prepared and found to express the X-linked genes G6PD and HGPRT, and to lack αGal and PGK. By combining this information with that which can be obtained from other X-autosome translocations, the relative location of the various X-linked loci should soon be known.

Somatic cell hybridization can also be used to analyze regulatory genes. This may ultimately prove to be its most important role, since no other means of analyzing regulatory genes presently exists. One of the most recent and interesting observations is that of Croce *et al.*[20] who report the behavior of tyrosine aminotransferase (TAT) in hybrids derived from human fibroblasts and rat hepatoma cells. TAT is not found when the human X chromosome is present but reappears when the human X is lost. Since TAT is present in the rat hepatoma parental cells and absent in the human fibroblast parental cells, these findings are interpreted as evidence for an X-linked gene(s) which inhibits expression of the rat TAT gene.

Somatic cell hybridization can be used to analyze the genetic basis of any cellular process for which an established cell line genetically defective in that process can be prepared. The recent development of a cell line defective in ribosomal RNA maturation[21] accentuates the variety of genetic events subject to study by cell hybridization. It is evident that the next few years will bring about an extraordinary increase in our knowledge of the human chromosome map.

REFERENCES

1. F.H. Ruddle, *Adv. Hum Genet. 3*, 173, 435, 1972.

2. F.H. Ruddle, *Nature 242*, 165, 1973.

3. K.-H. Grzeschik, *Humangenetik 19*,1, 1973.

4. M.C. Weiss and H. Green, *Proc. Nat. Acad. Sci. 58*, 1104, 1967.

5. J.H. Renwick, *Nature 234*, 475, 1971.

6. B. Watson, I.P. Gormley, S.E. Gardiner, H.J. Evans and H. Harris, *Exp. Cell Res. 75*, 401, 1972.

7. B. Bakay, C.M. Croce, H. Koprowski and W.L. Nyhan, *Proc. Nat. Acad. Sci. 70*, 1998, 1973.

8. C.M. Croce, B. Bakay, W.L. Nyhan and H. Koprowski, *Proc. Nat. Acad. Sci. 70*, 2590, 1973.

9. L.R. Weitkamp, S.A. Guttormsen and R.M. Greendyke, *Amer. J. Hum. Genet. 23*, 462, 1971.

10. A. Westerveld and P. Meera Khan, *Nature 236*, 30, 1972.

11. N. Van Cong, C. Billardon, J.-Y. Picard, J. Feingold and J. Frézal, *C.R. Acad. Sci. 272*, 485, 1971.

12. P.J.L. Cook, J. Noades, D.A. Hopkinson, E.B. Robson and T.E. Cleghorn, *Ann. Hum. Genet. 35*, 239, 1972.

13. F. Ruddle, F. Ricciuti, F.A. McMorris, J. Tischfield, R. Creagan, G. Darlington and T. Chen, *Science 176*, 1429, 1972.

14. V.C. Nguyen, C. Billardon, R. Reboutcet, C.L.B. de Kaoel, J.-Y. Picard, D. Weil and J. Frézal, *Ann. de Genetique 15*, 213, 1972.

15. G.A. Bruns and P.S. Gerald, Unpublished data.

16. E. Giblett, Personal communication.

17. Recommendations of the International Union of Biochemistry on the Nomenclature and Classification of Enzymes, 1964.

18. V.A. McKusick, Mendelian Inheritance in Man, 3rd Edition, The Johns Hopkins Press, Baltimore, 1971.

19. F. Ricciuti and F.H. Ruddle, *Nature 241*, 180, 1973.

20. C.M.Croce, G. Litwack and H. Koprowski, *Proc. Nat. Acad. Sci. 70*, 1268, 1973.

21. D. Toniolo, H.K. Meiss and C. Basilico, *Proc. Nat. Acad. Sci. 70*, 1273, 1973.

ADENOSINE DEAMINASE: GENETIC ASPECTS*

Eloise R. Giblett
C. Ronald Scott†
Shi-Han Chen†

I. The Genetic Polymorphism of Adenosine Deaminase

Adenosine deaminase is one of the several enzymes in the body which exhibit genetic polymorphism; i.e., they exist in two or more inherited structural forms with population frequencies greater than would be expected on the basis of mutation alone. For convenience, the minimum frequency indicative of polymorphism is set at one percent.

Harris and his colleagues[1] conducted a search for human genetic polymorphisms among more or less randomly chosen enzymes demonstrable by specific staining after starch gel electrophoresis. They found that about a third of the enzymes tested were polymorphic, including adenosine deaminase (ADA). This enzyme catalyzes the hydrolytic deamination of adenosine, producing inosine and ammonia. ADA activity is present in several body tissues but the highest levels are in the small bowel, spleen and red cells. In the technique devised for ADA staining,[2] the inosine formed is converted by nucleoside phosphorylase to hypoxanthine, which is then oxidized by xanthine oxidase. This reaction is coupled to the reduction of MTT, producing an insoluble dark blue formazan visible at the sites of ADA activity.

The three electrophoretic patterns shown in Figure 1 are those initially observed,[2] the phenotypes (ADA 1, 2 and 2-1) representing homozygosity and heterozygosity for two allelic genes, ADA^1 and ADA^2, at the autosomal structural locus. The frequency of ADA^1 is around 0.95 in most populations, although there is some geographic variation. There are also several rare variants of ADA with characteristic appearance on electrophoresis. One of the most

*This work was supported by PHS grants AM 09745 and GM 15253 and a grant from the National Foundation.

†Departments of Pediatrics and Medicine, University of Washington School of Medicine, Seattle, Washington.

Adenosine   Deaminase

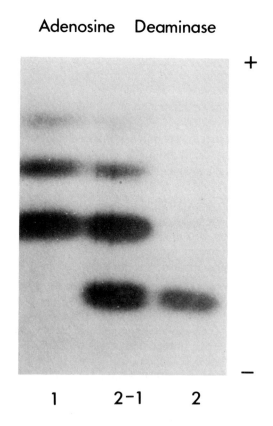

Figure 1. Starch gel electrophoretic patterns of three ADA phenotypes.

interesting was described by Hopkinson et al.[3] in an English family. Some members had the ADA 1, 2 and 2-1 phenotypes but others had an unusual electrophoretic pattern, designated as ADA 3-1. This pattern had the isozymes of ADA 1 plus an additional very faint band with a migration rate similar to that of the major isozyme of ADA 2. Inheritance studies showed that some members were heterozygous for either the ADA^1 or ADA^2 allele and a third allele, ADA^3, having a product with greatly reduced catalytic activity. No homozygotes for ADA^3 were found and, although this family did have a history of recurrent spontaneous abortion, there was no evidence that the unusual ADA phenotype was causally related.

II. The Discovery of ADA Deficiency Associated with CID

In our laboratories, several populations were studied for their ADA gene frequencies,[4] and ADA typing was included along with that of other enzymes in a battery of tests performed for human genetic studies. In June 1972, we were asked by Dr. Meuwissen to determine the genetic markers of a child who had severe combined immunodeficiency disease (CID) and was a candidate for possible bone marrow grafting. When this child's red cell hemolysate was tested for ADA phenotype, no isozyme bands could be seen. She was the product of a consanguineous mating and both of her parents had the isozymes characteristic of the ADA 1 phenotype, but with reduced staining intensity. Spectrophotometric assay confirmed the lack of measurable red cell ADA activity in the child and about half-normal levels in her parents.

Shortly thereafter, we obtained blood specimens from an unrelated girl in Detroit, who also had severe immune deficiency. The ADA phenotypes and catalytic activities of this patient and her parents were virtually identical with those of the Albany patient. It therefore appeared very probable that both sets of parents were heterozygous and their affected daughters were homozygous for a "silent" allele at the ADA structural locus with either no protein product or else a catalytically inactive or structurally unstable product. Furthermore, the association of ADA deficiency with CID in two unrelated children seemed very unlikely to be fortuitous.

III. Verifying the Existence of a "Silent" Allele

A description of these two cases,[5] published in November 1972, was quickly followed by a letter from Copenhagen[6] describing a third case of particularly severe CID and ADA deficiency with apparently reduced ADA levels in the parents. Soon afterwards, a male infant in Seattle died with CID, and he, too, was found to have ADA deficiency.[7] This child had many family members and their red cells were tested for ADA phenotype and catalytic activity.[8] As shown in an abbreviated pedigree (Figure 2), it was possible to assign their probable ADA genotypes on the basis of these tests. In the apparent carriers of the "silent" allele, tentatively called ADA^0, enzyme activity ranged from 14 to 24 units per gm hemoglobin. In the presumed non-carriers, the level ranged from 34 to 37, except for the sister of the propositus. Her value of 51.5 was much higher than the mean of 36 ± 6.5 found in 22 unrelated normal subjects but did not exceed the highest level in that group of people.

Further evidence for a "silent" allele was also provided by this family. II-2, with ADA 1, had a child (III-2) with ADA 2, indicating that both mother and daughter were carriers of an ADA gene with no visible product. The low enzyme activity in their red cells supplied further support for this conclusion.

IV. Clinical and Genetic Heterogeneity

As noted elsewhere in this symposium, several additional cases of CID with ADA deficiency have been found in this country and in Europe. However, one child has been reported to have red cell ADA deficiency without any clinical evidence of immune deficiency.[9] This child is a native of the South African Kalahari region. His ADA deficiency was first detected in 1971 during a routine study of genetic markers in South African Bushmen. Although starch gel electrophoresis of his red cell hemolysate revealed no ADA activity and the ADA isozymes of his father and sister had reduced activity, this boy had no history of recurrent infections and he appeared clinically well. He is now twelve years old and a recent test for red cell ADA gave the same results.[9] His lymphocyte count and immunoglobulin levels were in the normal range, as were his anti-A and anti-B isohemagglutinin titers. However, his skin reaction to PPD was very weak and there was no reaction to candida or Streptokinase/Streptodornase, suggesting the possibility of some impairment of cellular immunity.

This challenging case, as well as the fairly wide range in clinical severity found in the other children with ADA deficiency, is best explained by genetic and environmental heterogeneity. This so-called "silent" ADA gene has a low frequency and probably represents several different ADA genes at the structural locus for the enzyme. Those ADA deficient children who are the products of consanguineous matings are very likely to be homozygous for one of these rare alleles. However, the affected children in families without consanguinity are more likely to be "doubly heterozygous" for two different defective alleles at this locus. The variability in clinical manifestations undoubtedly reflects not only differences of this kind but also interactions with the total genome

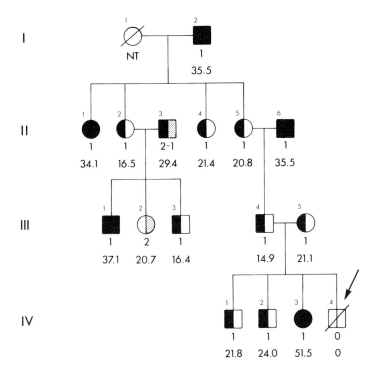

Figure 2. Pedigree of a family with an **ADA** deficient member. The numbers below each family member indicate the **ADA** electrophoretic phenotype (1, 2, 2-1 or 0) and the level of red cell activity in units per gm hemoglobin. The **ADA** genes are represented by black for *ADA1*, stippled for *ADA2* and white for *ADA0*.

107

in any given individual, as well as environmental factors.

V. An Alternative Genetic Hypothesis

At the time of our original report,[5] we proposed as an alternative genetic mechanism that the absence of ADA might be only a marker for the disease, rather than the cause of it. This suggestion was based on a report[10] that the locus for the red cell form of ADA might be genetically linked to the HL-A locus. The major histocompatibility locus in both mice and guinea pigs is very closely linked to the Ir genes which control the cellular immune response to specific antigens.[11] Thus, it seemed possible that the children with CID and ADA deficiency might be homozygous for a small chromosomal deletion involving the Ir genes and only incidentally including the ADA locus.

This hypothesis now seems to be quite unlikely. First of all, it would be a remarkable coincidence for the same, or a very similar, deletion to occur on a sufficient number of occasions in unrelated individuals to cause both CID and ADA deficiency in over a dozen children from different families. Secondly, recent evidence has placed the structural locus of red cell ADA on chromosome 20, while that of HL-A is probably on chromosome 6.[12] Thus, the linkage between the two loci now seems highly unlikely.

VI. The Number of ADA Loci

If the inherited deficiency of ADA does indeed act, according to classical models, as an inborn error blocking some essential metabolic step, it becomes necessary to determine which of the cells involved in the immune response are involved and how they are adversely affected. These questions are complicated by the possibility that ADA may have more than one structural gene locus. Edwards *et al.*[13] showed that extracts of various tissues contained several apparently tissue-specific isozymes not present in red cells, suggesting that there might be as many as four or five ADA loci. However, the elegant experiments of Dr. Rochelle Hirschhorn (described elsewhere in this Symposium) very strongly support a single ADA locus with tissue-specific alteration of the ADA gene product.

VII. ADA Isozymes in Lymphocytes and Fibroblasts

Both laboratory and clinical findings indicate that lack of ADA activity does not cause major alterations in the non-immune functions of the body and that the cell most likely to be adversely affected is the lymphocyte. When extracts of normal lymphocytes are subjected to electrophoresis and stained for ADA

108

activity, they always contain the isozymes corresponding to those of the individual's red cells. In addition, there is often a slower moving band of variable intensity which has the same mobility, regardless of red cell phenotype.[14] The isozyme pattern of cultured fibroblasts is very similar to that of lymphocytes.

Drs. Cooper and Keightley generously sent us some fibroblasts cultured from the skin of their Birmingham patient with CID and ADA deficiency. We found that the ADA activity of an extract of these cells was too weak to be seen on starch gels. However, when the extract was concentrated, the typical slow-moving isozyme was faintly visible after prolonged incubation. In view of Dr. R. Hirschhorn's findings (q.v.), we believe that the very low level of ADA activity in the fibroblasts of this child reflects the production of the enzyme molecules which are altered either in specific activity or structural stability.

VIII. Prenatal Diagnosis of ADA Deficiency

One of us (Shi-Han Chen) has recently measured the ADA activity per gram of protein in cultured fibroblasts derived from 26 normal subjects and found a range of 6.4 to 34 units, with a mean of 14.6 $\pm$ 6.8 units. Cells obtained by amniocentesis from 20 pregnant women had very similar levels. Since the fibroblasts of affected children have virtually no enzyme activity, it seems very likely that the diagnosis of ADA deficiency can be made *in utero*.[15]

IX. The Possibility of Other Enzyme Defects in Immunodeficiency Diseases

We have found that several children with combined immune deficiency have normal or elevated levels of ADA, as do children with other inherited diseases of immunity, such as Wiscott-Aldrich syndrome and ataxia telangiectasia. Some of these children have also been tested for other enzymes of purine and pyrimidine metabolism, including PRPP synthetase, nucleoside phosphorylase, adenylate kinase and guanylate kinase. So far, these enzymes have not shown marked reduction in activity or altered electrophoretic mobility. Nevertheless, because there is a long and growing list of enzyme deficiencies which alter the structural or functional integrity of various cells in the body, we feel confidant that other enzymes besides ADA are vital for normal lymphocyte function. It follows, then, that ADA deficiency is only the first of a series of enzyme defects which eventually will be found to cause inherited diseases of the immune system.

REFERENCES

1. H. Harris and D.A. Hopkinson, *Ann. Hum. Genet. 36,* 9, 1972.

2. N. Spencer, D.A. Hopkinson and H. Harris, *Ann. Hum. Genet. 32,* 9, 1968.

3. D.A. Hopkinson, P.J.L. Cook and H. Harris, *Ann. Hum. Genet. 32,* 361, 1969.

4. J.C. Detter, G. Stamatoyannopoulos, E.R. Giblett and A.G. Motolsky, *J. Med. Genet. 7,* 356, 1970.

5. E.R. Giblett, J.E. Anderson, F. Cohen, B. Pollara and H.J. Meuwissen, *Lancet II,* 1067, 1972.

6. J. Dissing and B. Knudsen, *Lancet II,* 1316, 1972.

7. J. Yount, P.Nichols, H.D. Ochs, S.P. Hammar, C.R. Scott, S.-H. Chen, E.R. Giblett and R.J. Wedgwood, *J. Pediat.* (In press)

8. S.-H. Chen, C.R. Scott and E.R. Giblett, *Am. J. Hum. Genet.* (In press)

9. T. Jenkins, *Lancet II,* 736, 1973.

10. J.H. Edwards, F.H. Allen, K.P. Glenn, L.U. Lamm and E.B. Robson, *in* Histocompability Testing, 1972, Munksgaard, Copenhagen, p. 745, 1973.

11. B. Benacerraf and H.O. McDevitt, *Science 175,* 273, 1972.

12. J.A. Tischfield, R.P. Creagan, E. Nichols and F.H. Ruddle, *Am. Soc. Hum. Genet.* 25th annual meeting, abstract, p. 80a, 1973.

13. Y.H. Edwards, D.A. Hopkinson and H. Harris, *Ann. Hum. Genet. 35,* 207, 1971.

14. H. Wüst, *Hum. Hered. 21,* 607, 1971.

15. S.-H. Chen and C.R. Scott, *Amer. Soc. Hum. Genet.* 25th annual meeting, abstract p. 21a, 1973.

STUDIES OF THE NATURE OF MULTIPLE ELECTROPHORETIC BANDS OF ADENOSINE DEAMINASE

Newton Ressler

An increasing interest in the genetic aspects of human adenosine deaminase (ADA) isozymes has been correlated with the detection of patients having both adenosine deaminase deficiency and impairment of cellular immunity.[1,2] Electrophoretic procedures have been fundamental for such studies. Since multiple bands could be due to a variety of causes,[3] those specific for multiple ADA bands might be especially important.

A systematic procedure for the determination of multiple bands has recently been described.[3] Some aspects of this approach which may be relevant to the study of the isozymes of ADA will be discussed in this communication.

Some Relevant Causes of Multiple Bands

Table 1 illustrates some of the possible reasons why an enzyme such as adenosine deaminase could exhibit multiple bands. Different primary structures could be associated with alleles, duplicate enzymes or separate genes.[4] It should always be kept in mind that differences in primary structure can occur without differences in mobility.

If the effective charge of a portion of the enzyme molecules is altered due to ligand binding or altered groups, different bands due to charge isomers could then result (i.e., bands due to the original and to the altered molecules). The isozymes of lactic dehydrogenase provide an illustrative example of such charge isomers. The well known isozymes of human lactic dehydrogenase are illustrated in the diagram of Fig. 1 by the 5 lines on the left (i.e., B_4, B_3A, B_2A_2, BA_3 and A_4). The horizontal lines on the right illustrate the type of pattern which is commonly used as evidence for the synthesis of two, slightly different, types of A subunits. Such patterns have been observed with a small proportion of hemolysates of human erythrocytes, for example.[5]

It has been observed, however, that by treating certain human tissues, which originally exhibited only the five single isozymes on the left of Fig. 1, with formaldehyde, the same pattern or regularly increasing sub-bands as on the

111

TABLE 1

Some Common Causes of Multiple Bands

---

1. Genetic: different primary structures

2. Multiple forms of the same enzyme molecule

   a) charge isomers

   b) size isomers

   c) conformationsl isomers

3. Interactions or artifacts

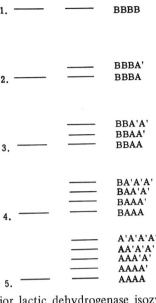

Fig. 1. The five major lactic dehydrogenase isozymes are illustrated by the horizontal lines on the left. The sub-bands, when two types of A subunits A and A′) are present, are shown on the right.

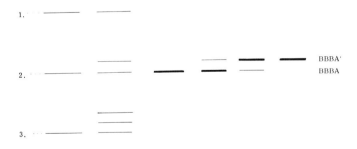

Fig. 2. The first three major isozymes are on the left. The second column illustrates sub-bands in these enzymes after formaldehyde treatment of whole tissue. The third column shows isolated isozyme 2, without treatment. The remaining aliquots of isolated isozyme 2 were treated (from left to right) with increasing concentrations of formaldehyde.

right of Fig. 1 can be obtained.[6] Single bands in the untreated tissue were isolated by preparative electrophoresis and different portions were treated with increasing concentrations of formaldehyde. As illustrated in the diagram of Fig. 2 for isozyme 2, the relative proportion of activity in the most anodal sub-band increased with formaldehyde concentration, from 0% for no formaldehyde to 100% at the highest concentration.[7] The results would appear to indicate that formaldehyde reacts with some of the A but not the B subunits. The A subunits which have, and those which have not, reacted with formaldehyde would then constitute two electrophoretic species of A subunits.

With two types of A subunits, whether due either to the synthesis of different primary structures or to changes in a portion of the molecules after synthesis, the electrophoretic pattern of increasing sub-bands would be the same. If the resistance of an enzyme molecule to *in vitro* or *in vivo* alterations after synthesis were affected by other inherited metabolic variations, false impressions about the genetic control of the enzyme could easily be obtained.

It should be noted that the reaction of a ligand with a portion of the enzyme molecules could have another effect in addition to or instead of altering the mobility. Certain reagents, for example, might cause an inhibition of the A subunits with which they react. In this case, instead of sub-bands, there would be progressive inhibition of activity, ranging from zero for isozyme 1 to a maximum for isozyme 5. In the case of serum lactic dehydrogenase, this type of effect may be obtained under certain conditions by freezing or heating.[8] Such changes may again mimic changes in the electrophoretic patterns which are due to genetic factors (i.e., in which the mutation of an enzyme subunit or molecule results in a loss of activity[9]).

The final criteria for the distinction of changes after synthesis from changes in primary structure is, of course, the determination of the primary structure. However, the ability to convert, *in vitro,* one form of an enzyme to another one, may often provide a simple means of demonstrating multiple forms of a given molecule as a cause of multiple bands (see below).

In the case of tissue specific bands or characteristic electrophoretic patterns for particular tissue types, the multiple bands may still be due to different forms of the same enzyme molecule. Various human tissues, for example, have been shown to exhibit characteristic patterns of glyceraldehyde-3-phosphate dehydrogenase activity.[10] As illustrated in Fig. 3, essentially all of the activity in supernatants of homogenates prepared from heart, skeletal muscle or liver, was consistently restricted to a single, less anodal "slow band". In other tissues, such as spleen, adrenal, thyroid or lung, all, or the largest portion, of the activity was always exhibited in a more anodal "fast band". In kidney supernatants, the activity was about equally divided between the fast and slow bands.

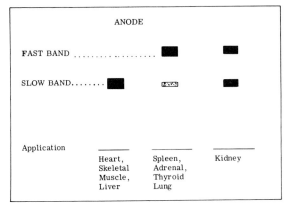

Fig. 3. Characteristic glyceraldehyde-3-phosphate dehydrogenase bands for different types of tissues.

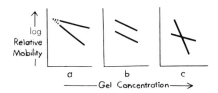

Fig. 4. Distinction of 2 proteins which differ in size or charge as described by Hedrick and Smith.[13] In "a" the 2 proteins differ in size but not charge, in "b" they differ in charge but not size, while in "c" they differ in both.

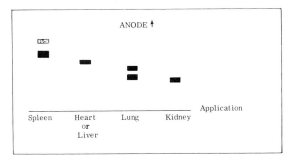

Fig. 5. ADA bands exhibited by different types of tissues.

115

Despite the fact that the type of pattern consistently depended upon the type of tissue, evidence has been obtained that the two bands represent different forms of the same enzyme molecule. Either the fast band or the slow band could be converted, *in vitro*, into the other in a reversible manner. A fraction from homogenates favored the formation of the fast band and inhibited activity. The fast band was converted into the slow band by additions of ADP or NAD^+, which tend to increase glycolytic activity. Since NAD^+ is also known to alter the conformation of glyceraldehyde-3-phosphate dehydrogenase,[11] such electrophoretic patterns could provide an approach toward the study of conformational changes in the control of enzyme activity.[10] The possibility that particular bands can represent forms of an enzyme which depend upon tissue specific, cellular environments can relate to the interpretation of various other enzyme patterns. Besides charge or conformational isomers, the same considerations may apply to size isomers such as those of glutamic dehydrogenase, for example.[12]

An effective method of detecting such isomers, in addition to the technique of interconversions, is the variation in starch or polyacrylamide gel concentration. The method described by Hedrick and Smith permits the distinction of size isomers, Fig. 4a; charge isomers, Fig. 4b; or proteins which differ in both, Fig. 4c.[13] The slope in Fig. 4a can be directly related to the molecular weight by the analysis of various "standard proteins" of known molecular weight. If the gel concentration is low enough, the size isomers are no longer distinguished. With molecules of the same size but different charges, the slopes are the same and the lines are parallel.

Isozyme Patterns of ADA

The considerations described above illustrate some of those which might be of use in the interpretation of electrophoretic patterns which have been obtained in the case of ADA. Preliminary investigations of adenosine deaminase in human tissues by the present author[14] can serve as an example. Human autopsy samples were homogenized with 1.5 ml of water per g wet weight. The latter were applied to starch gels (9.6 g starch/100 ml) prepared with a Tris-citrate buffer, pH 7.0. After electrophoresis, bands with ADA activity were determined by a modification of the method of Tully and Walsh.[15]

Samples of spleen, heart, liver, lung and kidney were investigated. Several dozen samples were studied and it was found that the same type of tissue consistently exhibited the same type of pattern as illustrated in Fig. 5. The mobilities of the most intense bands were greatest for homogenates of spleen, less for heart or liver, still less for lung and the least for kidney.

Most of the activity of the spleen samples was exhibited in two distinct bands. When a portion of the spleen homogenate had been heated at 60° for

116

30 minutes, the activity of the forward band increased, while that of the more slowly migrating band decreased, Fig. 6. If portions of spleen and lung homogenates were separated at a starch gel concentration of 15 g/100 ml (instead of 9.6 g/100 ml), the relative mobility of the lung sample decreased considerably more than that of the spleen at the higher starch gel concentration (i.e., the lung sample had a greater retardation coefficient), Fig. 7. An additional, more anodal, spleen band was resolved at the higher gel concentration in the heated sample.

Discussion

The association of the increase in activity of the forward spleen band with the decrease in activity of the slower band, after heating (Fig. 6), would suggest that the rear band is converted into the forward one. Previously, Cory, Weinbaum and Suhadolnik also demonstrated an apparent conversion of a calf serum band into the faster one by heat.[16] A similar shift of activity from the slower to the faster isozymes of red cell lysates was shown by Spencer, Hopkinson and Harris[17] to be caused by storage at 4° C, or by addition of oxidized glutathione. In some cases more anodal bands developed (analogous to that in Fig. 7, above). These effects were reversed by 2-mercaptoethanol. Comparable results were subsequently obtained by Edwards, Hopkinson and Harris with red cell-like bands in a number of different tissues.[18] However, no activity shifts were found with other, more slowly migrating bands.

ADA is known to contain a reactive-SH group, which isn't required for activity.[19] The above results could be accounted for in a simple manner if either heating, storage or oxidized glutathione increased the extent of reaction of this -SH group and if this, in turn, resulted in an increase in mobility. The reversal of the anodal activity shifts by 2-mercaptoethanol indicates that these particular bands represent different forms of the same molecule. These more anodal spleen or red blood cell bands have molecular weights in the neighborhood of 34,000.[18]

In the case of the more cathodal bands such as those in lung or kidney, the greater retardation coefficient illustrated in Fig. 7 and the gel filtration experiments of Edwards, Hopkinson and Harris[18] both indicate that the molecular weights are greater. In the latter experiments, values around 280,000 or 435,000 were obtained for different bands. Murphy, Brady and Boggust had previously found molecular weights of 251,000 and 34,000 by gel filtration of rabbit duodenum extracts.[20]

The considerations discussed above would suggest that it is not necessary to exclude the possibility that all of the ADA bands are due to different forms of the same enzyme molecule. Edwards, Hopkinson and Harris did consider that

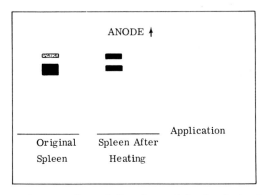

Fig. 6. Apparent conversion of the slower into the faster ADA bands in spleen by heating.

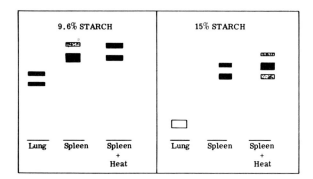

Fig. 7. Lung, spleen and heated spleen homogenates, separated in 9.6 g of starch per 100 ml on the left (as in Figs. 5 and 6), and in 15.0 g of starch per 100 ml on the right.

one possibility consistent with their results would be that all of the larger ADA molecules are due to aggregates of the smaller, red cell ADA. This possibility would depend upon the abolition, by the aggregation, of sulphhydryl group reactivity and of the mobility differences between the red cell bands. It should be noted, however, that if differences in a reactive-SH group are involved in the differences between the red cell band mobilities, and if this -SH group becomes tied up during aggregation, these characteristics of the "polymer" bands would be explained. Murphy, Brady and Boggust did observe, during re-runs of isolated gel filtration bands, that some of the 150,000 molecular weight ADA molecules dissociated into smaller sizes[20] while Hoagland and Fisher found that the smaller 31,000 molecular weight chicken duodenal enzyme tended to aggregate in a concentrated solution.[19]

It would appear that additional electrophoretic studies in which such techniques as interconversions, or the use of a number of different gel concentrations for the distinction of size and charge isomers, could help to provide further characterization of the various human ADA bands. Such types of investigations illustrate how the elimination of variables by their specific study can lead to a more dynamic and complete picture of the molecules than the relatively limited information obtainable from a single run under one set of electrophoretic conditions.[3]

REFERENCES

1. E.R. Giblett, J.E. Anderson, F. Cohen, B. Pollara and H.J. Meuwissen, *Lancet II*, 1067, 1972.

2. J. Dissing and J.B. Knudsen, *Hum. Hered. 20*, 178, 1970.

3. N. Ressler, *Anal. Biochem. 51*, 589, 1973.

4. N.O. Kaplan, *Ann. N.Y. Acad. Sci. 151*, 382, 1968.

5. A.P. Kraus and C.L. Neeley, Jr., *Science 145*, 595, 1964.

6. N. Ressler and C. Tuttle, *Nature 210*, 1268, 1966.

7. N. Ressler, *Nature 215*, 284, 1967.

8. J.F. Kachmar, *in* Fundamentals of Clinical Chemistry, N.W. Tietz (Ed.), W.B. Saunders Co., Philadelphia, 1970.

9. C.R. Shaw, Brookhaven Symposium in Biology, No. 17, 117, 1964.

10. N. Ressler and S. Lee, *Biochem. J. 119*, 85, 1970.

11. H. Durchslag, G. Puchwein, O. Kratty, I Schuster and K. Kirschner, *F.E.B.S., Lett. 4,* 75, 1969.

12. N. Ressler and K. Stitzer, *Biochim. Biophys. Acta 146,* 1, 1967.

13. J.L. Hedrick and A.J. Smith, *Arch. Biochem. Biophys. 126,* 155, 1968.

14. N. Ressler, *Clin. Chim. Acta 24,* 247, 1969.

15. T.G. Brady and C.J. O'Donovan, *Comp. Biochem. Physiol. 14,* 101, 1965.

16. J.C. Cory, G. Weinbaum and R.J. Suhadolnik, *Arch. Biochem. Biophys. 118,* 418, 1967.

17. N. Spencer, D.A. Hopkinson and H. Harris, *Ann. Hum. Genet. 32,* 9, 1968.

18. Y.H. Edwards, D.A. Hopkinson and H. Harris, *Ann. Hum. Genet. 35,* 207, 1971.

19. V.D. Hoagland and J.R. Fisher, *J. Biol. Chem. 242,* 4341, 1967.

20. P.M. Murphy, T.G. Brady and W.A. Boggust, *Biochim. Biophys. Acta 188,* 341, 1969.

ADENOSINE DEAMINASE DEFICIENCY: GENETIC AND METABOLIC IMPLICATIONS*

Rochelle Hirschhorn

The finding of an inherited absence of adenosine deaminase associated with disease[1,2,3] has given us a tool with which to explore and clarify several different aspects of normal and abnormal human development. First, it allows us to examine the genetic and molecular interrelationships of the different forms of adenosine deaminase. An understanding of this relationship becomes important for proper prenatal diagnosis of this disease. Second, this experiment of nature may give us information as to the normal differentiation of lymphocytes into immunocompetent cells and, lastly, this disease may well make apparent new pathways of normal purine and pyrimidine biosynthesis.

I would like to discuss some of our studies; primarily those relating to the relationship between the different isozymes of ADA but also touching upon these other aspects. Just to briefly review the different forms or isozymes of adenosine deaminase; in red blood cells, adenosine deaminase activity is exhibited by an enzyme protein of approximately 35,000 molecular weight which migrates relatively rapidly on starch gel. This protein is apparently modified after translation to give rise to two secondary enzyme bands. This results in the typical triple banded pattern which very conveniently allows us to identify what is called the RBC isozyme. This protein is also polymorphic in that there are inherited differences in electrophoretic mobility in different individuals which provide another way to mark the RBC isozyme[4,5] but they also contain several other tissue isozymes. This is presented diagrammatically in Figure 1. On the right we see the RBC isozymes shaded. The tissue isozymes are represented next to the RBC isozymes for the purposes of clarity. The nomenclature suggested by Edwards et al. will be used.[4] The most common of the tissue isozymes (labeled d) is seen in most tissues as well as in fibroblasts and circulating T lymphocytes. This isozyme has a molecular

*Aided by a grant from the National Institutes of Health (A1 10343).
** Rochelle Hirschhorn is a recipient of an N.I.H. Research Career Development Award (A1 70254).

weight of over 200,000. The slower isozyme (labeled e) is typical of kidney and intestines and has a molecular weight of over 440,000. Two minor isozymes (labeled b and c) are variably expressed in most tissues and have the same molecular weight as the d isozyme. These "tissue specific" isozymes do not demonstrate the polymorphism observed in the RBC form of the enzyme in that they do not vary in electrophoretic mobility in individuals of differing ADA RBC phenotypes. Therefore, the several tissue specific isozymes are considered to be determined at one or more separate genetic loci not allelic with the locus for RBC ADA.

The finding of an inherited absence of red blood cell ADA[1,2,3] has allowed us to examine the genetic interrelationship of these ADA isozymes. We have had the opportunity to examine stored tissues from one of these patients (T. Ha)[1] which has been extremely informative.[6]

Extracts of normal liver contained two major isozymes, one with a mobility between that of the first and second band of the RBC ADA isozymes (isozyme "a") and a second band migrating less rapidly with a mobility similar to that of a band seen in lymphocytes and fibroblasts (Fig. 1) (isozyme "d"). It can be seen in channel 2, that extracts of the patient's liver did not contain either isozyme. Normal kidney extracts (channel 3) revealed one major area of activity with a mobility overlapping and slower than that of the "d" isozyme (isozymes "d" and "e"). The patænt's kidney (channel 4) again contained no activity. Normal heart homogenates (channel 5) demonstrated the slower mobility "d" isozyme and the intermediate mobility large molecular weight tissue isozyme "b-c" as well as the RBC ADA isozymes. These isozymes were also absent in extracts of the patient's heart. Normal splenic homogenates (Fig. 2, channel 2) showed predominantly an RBC ADA pattern in this individual (who has a 2-1 phenotype) as did muscle. Normal intestinal extracts, revealed areas of activity in the "a,b,c,d and e" zones. Neither muscle, spleen nor intestines of the patient revealed any activity. A lymphoid line of ADA RBC 2-1 phenotype is seen in channel 7 for reference.

To summarize, when homogenates of kidney, liver, intestines, spleen, heart and muscle of the affected child were subjected to electrophoresis in parallel with the homogenates from normal tissues. The "red blood cell" isozymes, as seen in Figures 1 and 2, were absent. This confirms the earlier conclusion that the gene controlling transcription of the protein "RBC-ADA" is expressed in non-hematopoietic tissue.[4] However, contrary to prior expectations, none of the tissue specific isozymes of adenosine deaminase could be detected in any tissue examined from this child, although they were easily visualized in normal tissue.

It is unlikely that the absence of these isozymes was due to loss of enzyme activity during storage at $-70^{\circ}C$ for four months prior to examination since

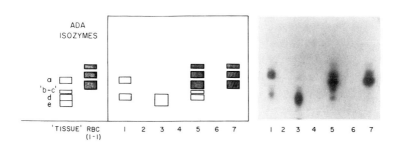

Fig. 1. Tissue homogenates were subjected to starch gel electrophoresis and stained for adenosine deaminase activity.[2] The various isozymes found in different tissues are represented diagrammatically using a previously suggested nomenclature.[1] The isozymes which are specific for RBC's but present in other tissues are indicated in the diagram as shaded areas. Channel 1 contained normal liver, channel 2 = patient's liver, channel 3 = normal kidney, channel 5 = normal heart, channel 6 = patient's heart, channel 7 contains a normal lymphoid line of RBC ADA phenotype 1-1 for reference.

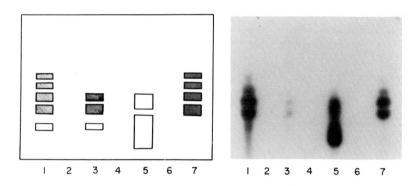

Fig. 2. Tissues were treated in the same manner as those in Figure 1 but were obtained from an individual of ADA 2-1 phenotype. Channel 1 contains normal intestines, channel 2 = patient's intestines, channel 3 = normal muscle, channel 4 = patient's muscle, channel 5 = normal intestines, channel 6 = patient's intestines, channel 7 = normal lymphoid line of RBC ADA 2-1 phenotype.

Conversion of 'RBC' ADA Isozymes to 'Tissue Specific' ADA Isozymes

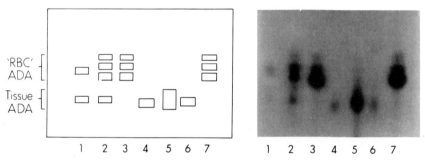

Fig. 3. Ten microliters of various dilutions of the lymphoid line extracts, which contained only the "red blood cell" isozyme, were incubated with 40 microliters of the different tissue extracts. The mixtures were incubated at room temperature for five hours prior to electrophoresis. Channel 1 = normal liver, channel 2 = lymphocytoid cells and liver extract from an ADA deficient child (see channel 2, Fig. 1), channel 3 = lymphocytoid line alone, channel 4 = normal kidney, channel 5 = lymphocytoid line and kidney extract of ADA deficient child (see Fig. 1, channel 4), channel 6 = normal fibroblast, channel 7 = normal lymphocytoid lines.

ADA isozymes were still detectable in tissues of normals which had been stored either as homogenates or as whole tissues for up to six months at -20°C. Matching samples from the normal and immunodeficient individuals contained equal amounts of protein (as determined by the method of Lowry) as well as equivalent amounts of two other enzyme activities, nucleoside phosphorylase[7] and adenylate kinase,[8] as visualized following starch gel electrophoresis. Fibroblasts from the patient were found to have no visible isozymes of adenosine deaminase activity. It thus appears that, in spite of the tissue to tissue variation in electrophoretic mobility of adenosine deaminase and the absence of any visible polymorphism, the different enzyme activities are controlled by a single structural genetic locus.

Several previous reports have suggested that large molecular weight (presumably tissue specific) and low molecular weight (presumably RBC) forms of ADA are structurally related. Thus, Ressler[9] observed that heating spleen homogenates at 60°C appeared to convert the slow (large molecular weight) ADA to the more rapidly migrating (presumably smaller) ADA. More recently, Akedo *et al.* have demonstrated that human tissues contain a heat labile molecule which when incubated with a low molecular weight (presumably RBC) ADA, cause its conversion to a large molecular weight form.[10,11] In preliminary experiments, we have been able to convert RBC ADA derived from lymphoid lines of different phenotypes to the several different tissue specific isozymes by incubating with extracts of tissue from this patient and normal individuals[12] (Fig. 3).

Some residual ability to metabolize adenosine appears to be retained in fibroblasts derived from this child.[13] This activity (if it is not simply endocytosed from serum used in culturing) may either represent an alternate pathway, the activity of a weak non-allelic isozyme which is not detected on electrophoresis or the residual activity of a genetically altered, very labile and/or inefficient ADA enzyme. It is well recognized that most cases of so-called genetically determined "absent" enzymes truly represent an altered protein (cross-reacting material) which may retain some residual activity. In fact, we have found an electrophoretic altered low activity mutant enzyme present in fibroblasts derived from four cases reported here and have extensively characterized this enzyme in the fibroblasts derived from a patient of Dr. F. Rosen.

The finding that all of the isozymes of ADA are controlled at the same genetic locus is of importance for the possible prenatal diagnosis of this illness. Fibroblasts from the same person vary with time as to whether they express the red cell isozyme, the tissue isozyme or both. We have observed that cultured normal amniotic cells also vary as to which isozyme they express. The ADA activity of amniotic cells can be easily assayed and is similar to or slightly higher than that of normal human fibroblasts. Moreover, since the structural unit of both of these isozymes is controlled by the same locus as that involved in ADA deficiency associated with severe combined immunodeficiency, prenatal diagnosis is possible no matter which isozyme is expressed.[14]

Adenosine deaminase would appear to have a unique importance for the development of the immunocompetent lymphoid cell. When peripheral blood lymphocytes are stimulated to enter a proliferative phase by addition of mitogens such as PHA, they undergo a series of complex metabolic alterations. These changes presumably mirror the alterations in cellular metabolism during an *in vivo* cellular immune response.[15] In order to examine the possible role of ADA in the economy of the immune system, we have examined alterations in ADA isozymes after stimulation of lymphocytes by various mitogens.

When extracts of lymphocytes, which had previously been purified from other hematopoietic elements, were electrophoresed on starch gel and the adenosine deaminase activity visualized, two major areas of activity were evident. These cell preparations contained the polymorphic triple banded protein which is characteristic of red blood cells (RBC ADA) and a second isozyme of slower mobility at pH 6.5. This pattern remained constant over at least five days of tissue culture without PHA. When PHA was added to these lymphocyte preparations at the beginning of the culture period, this tissue specific isozyme became markedly diminished.

This alteration can be quantitated. Extracts of lymphocytes were applied to a Sephadex G 150 column which separates protein on the basis of size. It was found that the tissue specific isozyme of lymphocytes was of large molecular weight while the RBC isozymes emerged in fractions compatible with a molecular weight of 35,000. It can be seen that 35% of the total activity was present as tissue isozyme at the start of culture and a similar 24% after 72 hours without stimulation. However, if lymphocytes have been stimulated, only 8% of the ADA activity could be seen as tissue specific isozyme.[16]

Interestingly, while stimulation with Concanavalin A, presumably a T cell mitogen, also caused a decrease in tissue ADA, stimulation with PWM, presumably a B cell mitogen, did not cause a change in tissue isozymes, perhaps because B lymphocytes do not appear to contain tissue specific isozymes.[17]

The significance and importance of this alteration in isozyme pattern in the economy of the lymphoid cell might be related to differences in properties of the two forms of the enzyme. Two major differences[11,12] have been observed between the large and small forms of adenosine deaminase. The larger form is more heat stable whereas the smaller adenosine deaminase has a greater activity per mole of enzyme. Teleologically speaking, the shift from the tissue to the red cell form, seen in PHA stimulated lymphocytes, would provide an active although less stable enzyme without altering the rate of synthesis of that protein.

The need for adenosine deaminase in lymphocyte proliferation is perhaps reflected by some observations we made a number of years ago while studying the effect of cAMP on lymphocyte proliferation. Exogenous cAMP inhibits PHA induced lymphocyte proliferation. However, both adenosine and AMP are more effective on a mole per mole basis than is cAMP in inhibiting RNA, protein and DNA synthesis by stimulated lymphocytes.[18] This phenomenon has been elegantly explored and a possible mechanism offered by the studies of Dr. Howard Green, presented at this Symposium.

In summary, these studies demonstrate that the structural subunit of several of the tissue isozymes of adenosine deaminase appears to be controlled by the same genetic locus as that determining RBC ADA. This makes it feasible to perform prenatal diagnosis in this disease independent of which isozyme is expressed in amniotic cells.

These studies also demonstrate that stimulation of lymphocytes by PHA and Concanavalin A results in a loss of the tissue specific ADA. This alteration may represent a modulation of enzyme activity requisite for the more efficient handling of the potentially toxic metabolite, adenosine, and/or for providing for more efficient salvage of adenosine for increased purine and pyrimidine synthesis during proliferation of immunocompetent lymphocytes.

REFERENCES

1. E. Giblett, J. Anderson, F. Cohen, B. Pollara and H.J. Meuwissen, *Lancet II,* 1067, 1972.

2. J. Dissing and B. Knudsen, *Lancet II,* 1316, 1972.

3. H.H. Ochs, J.E. Yount, E.R. Giblett, S.H. Chen, C.R. Scott and R.J. Wedgwood, *Lancet I,* 1393, 1973.

4. Y.H. Edwards, D.A. Hopkinson and H. Harris, *Ann. Hum. Genet. 35,* 207, 1971.

5. N. Spencer, D.A. Hopkinson and H. Harris, *Ann. Hum. Genet. 32,* 9, 1968.

6. R. Hirschhorn, V. Levytska, H.J. Meuwissen and B. Pollara, *Nature, New Biol. 246,* 200, 1973.

7. Y.H. Edwards, D.A. Hopkinson and H. Harris, *Ann. Hum. Genet. 34,* 395, 1971.

8. R.A. Fildes and H. Narris, *Nature 209,* 261, 1966.

9.   N. Ressler, *Clin. Chim. Acta 24,* 147, 1969.

10.   K. Nishihara, S. Ishikawa, K. Shinkai and H. Akedo, *Biochim. Biophys. Acta 302,* 429, 1973.

11.   H. Akedo, H. Nishihara, K. Shinai, K. Komatsu and S. Ishikawa, *Biochim. Biophys. Acta 275,* 257, 1972.

12.   R. Hirschhorn and V. Levytska (submitted).

13.   H.J. Meuwissen (personal communication).

14.   R. Hirschhorn and N. Beratis, *Lancet II,* 1217, 1973.

15.   K. Hirschhorn and R. Hirschhorn, *in* Mechanisms of Cellular Immunity, S. Cohen and R. McClusky (Eds.), Interscience Pub. Div. of John Wiley and Sons (in press).

16.   R. Hirschhorn and V. Levytska, *J. Cell Immunol.* (in press).

17.   R. Hirschhorn and C. Bianco (unpublished observations).

18.   R. Hirschhorn, J. Grossman and G. Weissmann, *Proc. Soc. Exp. Biol. Med. 133,* 1361, 1970.

ADENOSINE DEAMINASE AND LYMPHOCYTE FUNCTION: BIOLOGICAL AND BIOCHEMICAL CONSIDERATIONS*

Bernard Pollara

The discovery that adenosine deaminase (ADA) deficiency is associated with combined immunodeficiency disease (CID) is another step in fulfilling the prediction that primary immunodeficiency syndromes would eventually be defined in terms of specific inborn errors of metabolism. Previously, our theories of pathogenesis of primary immune defects concentrated on the failures of development of central or peripheral lymphoid tissues at various levels of development. We must now reassess this view and reexamine our theories of the formation and development of the lymphoid system.

Although a number of patients with CID have been shown to lack ADA and, so far at least, no normal person has been shown to have comparable ADA deficiency, we cannot yet ascribe a cause-and-effect relationship to ADA deficiency and CID, but the repeated occurrence of these same defects in the same patients might be a clue to the role of purine metabolism in the development of lymphoid tissue.

Peterson, Cooper and Good's hypothesis[1] from the mid-60's represents the classical anatomical view of primary immunodeficiency. They proposed that a block at the level of a hypothetical lymphoid stem cell would give rise to the X-linked and the autosomal recessive forms of CID so that no cells would be available to be routed into T or B cell pathways of differentiation by the thymic and "bursal" influences. They accounted for selective aberrations of T or B cell development by defects further along the respective pathways of differentiation from the lymphoid stem cell.

We must now recast these concepts in biochemical terms to account for the association of ADA deficiency and CID and, perhaps, predict the type of biochemical lesion which characterizes CID patients with normal ADA levels.

Following the review of case histories of the CID-ADA deficient patients at the Workshop preceding this conference, we find:

*Supported in part by National Institutes of Health, Division of Research Resources, General Clinical Research Center, Grant 1-MO-RR00749.

1. Variable expression of T and B cell deficits, and

2. Variable involvement of other tissues, such as bone, pituitary and kidney. Thus, any satisfactory linking of ADA deficiency to the observed diseases has to account, on the one hand, for the primacy of the effects on lymphoid tissues, the more consistent effects on T than B cell development and, on the other hand, for the range of abnormalities of other organs.

One factor which may bear on this is the maternal influence on the fetus. The evidence is that ADA deficiency is an autosomal recessive condition and that, necessarily, both parents have a partial defect in purine metabolism. It is also likely, based on more detailed knowledge of enzyme defects in other metabolic diseases, that the defective enzymes themselves show biochemical variations. *In vitro* studies of lymphoid cell function early in human development have increasingly shown early maturation of immunologic capabilities: significant stimulation by allogeneic cells as early as the 11th week of development[2] and presence of B cell markers for IgM, IgA and IgG as early as the 12th week of fetal life.[3]

Maturation of the thymus has been studied in great detail. Cells with T cell characteristics enter the thymus as early as the eighth week of gestation; the thymic medullary areas are defined by the 12th and 13th weeks and the cortex and medulla are fully differentiated by the 21st week.[4] Lack of cortical medullary separation is characteristic of CID.

Concepts of B cell differentiation and function have also undergone revision in recent years. As noted, immunoglobulin markers may be detected as early as the 12th week. Four weeks later, immunoglobulin-secreting cells may be found.[3]

There is no indication that the ADA deficient form of CID represents a decline from more adequate function at birth except in the patient described by Giblett *et al.*[5] Most data suggest that the effects of the enzyme deficiency are manifest before birth, probably long before birth. The analysis by Huber and Kersey (this volume) of the state of differentiation of the thymus in ADA deficient patients supports this view. Thus, there is an interplay of the enzyme deficiency in the fetus, the partial enzyme deficiency in the mother and any ameliorating or modulating influences in the prenatal environment. The notion of immunologic stimulation of the fetus during normal prenatal development has been gaining acceptance and most of us believe that active antibody production occurs by antigens other than infectious agents. The nature of these stimuli and the response to them, whether T cell dependent or independent, might also modify the course of lymphoid development in the fetus with ADA deficiency.

In summary, genetic heterogeneity may play a role in the variable expression of ADA deficiency, both in the lymphoid tissues and in other organs. My present guess, however, is that the environmental cause(s) is the most important modifier of a small number of functionally defective enzymes. We should, therefore, study ADA deficient children from birth. In this connection, Meuwissen and Moore[6] have devised an ingenious screening test for ADA which may be used in the newborn. A thorough evaluation of mothers of affected infants, particularly relative to antigen exposure of the fetus, may offer some insights into the variable B and T cell dysfunction in ADA deficient children.

An animal model for CID and ADA deficiency would be helpful. Such a model may be at hand: McGuire *et al.*[7] have described CID in Arabian horses, and these animals are now being screened for ADA activity.

I should like to turn from these clinical considerations to one of the relationship between purine metabolism in the lymphoid and other tissues of these patients.

The effects of an enzyme deficiency may be secondary to the lack of a product, precursor accumulation or regulatory disturbance such as lack of feedback inhibition. Phenylketonuria, Fabry's disease and the Lesch-Nyhan syndrome respectively are examples of these effects.[8]

Two inborn errors of metabolism have been of interest in our attempt to define the nature of the association between ADA deficiency and CID: hereditary orotic aciduria, the only known inborn error affecting pyrimidine biosynthesis, and the Lesch-Nyhan syndrome, the first described inborn error of purine metabolism. Megaloblastic anemia is a cardinal feature of hereditary orotic aciduria but these patients are also lymphopenic and it is interesting that the first patient described with orotic aciduria died with an overwhelming varicella infection.[9]

The Lesch-Nyhan syndrome presents particular problems because it is not associated with immunologic deficiency or lymphopenia although it involves another step in purine recycling. There is unusual synthesis of purines *de novo* in the Lesch-Nyhan syndrome[10] but no evidence that this occurs in unstimulated lymphoid cells. Historically, the question of *de novo* purine synthesis in peripheral lymphocytes has not always been answered the same way. Recent work, using improved techniques of lymphocyte separation, suggests, however, that these cells only use purine recycling pathways, whereas cells stimulated with phytohemagglutinin synthesize the purine ring.[11] Studies on synchronized cultured lymphoid cell lines at various points in the cell cycle may help to resolve this problem.

Adenosine may be phosphorylated to adenosine monophosphate (AMP) or deaminated by ADA to inosine.[12] Adenosine is recycled to some extent following conversion first to inosine and then to hypoxanthine.[13] Hypoxanthine-guanine-phosphoribosyltransferase (HGPRT) converts hypoxanthine to

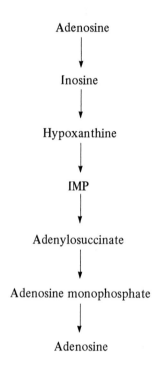

Fig. 1. Adapted from T.S. Chen, U. Ishii, C. Long and H.J. Green, *J. Cell Physiol. 81,* 315, 1873.

inosine monophosphate and subsequent reactions result in production of adenosine (Fig. 1). This has been called the adenosine cycle. Inosine kinase may be functional in PHA stimulated peripheral lymphoid cells, from both normal individuals and patients with Lesch-Nyhan syndrome.[14,15]

Interruption of the adenosine cycle at the point of conversion to inosine could saturate the adenosine kinase reactions and raise intracellular levels of ATP. This development may inhibit the conversion of orotic acid to uridine and cause the cells to die of pyrimidine starvation.[16] Levels of ATP, ADP and AMP have not yet been measured in lymphocytes from ADA deficient patients but in red cells of two such patients adenine nucleotides were not present in abnormal amounts.[17]

Thus, the precise role that ADA plays in the development and function of immunocompetent cells has yet to be established. Ultimately, our goal is to determine how the metabolic block resulting from the enzyme deficiency prevents normal lymphoid cell function and whether other enzyme defects are responsible for other immune deficiency syndromes. Careful studies of our patients will continue to give us, as in the past, further keys for our understanding of the immune system and mechanisms of host defense.

Our patients have once again provided us with a new perspective. It remains for us to capitalize on this new insight by defining the lymphoid system and immunity more accurately and thereby making it possible to devise effective forms of therapy.

REFERENCES

1. R.D.A. Peterson, M.D. Cooper and R.A. Good, *Amer. J. Med. 38,* 579. 1965.

2. M.C. Carr, D.P. Stites and H.H. Fudenberg, *Nature (New Biol.) 241,* 279, 1973.

3. A.R. Lawton, K.S. Self, S.A. Royal and M.D. Cooper, *Clin. Imm. and Immunopath. 1,* 84, 1973.

4. G. Goldstein and I.R. Mackay, The Human Thymus, Warren Green, Inc., St. Louis, 1969.

5. E.R. Giblett, J.E. Anderson, F. Cohen, B. Pollara and H.J. Meuwissen, *Lancet 2,* 1067, 1972.

6. E.C. Moore and H.J. Meuwissen, *J. Pediat.,* 1975 (in press).

7. T.C. McGuire and M.I. Poppie, *Infection and Immunity 272,* 8, 1973.

8.   J.B. Stanbury, J.B. Wyngaarden and D.S. Fredrickson (Eds.), The Metabolic Basis of Inherited Disease, McGraw-Hill, New York, p. 266, p. 663, p. 969, 1972.

9.   C.M. Hugulet, Jr., J.A. Bain, S. Rivers and R. Scoggins, *Blood 14,* 615, 1959.

10.   A.W. Wood, M.A. Becker and J.E. Seegmiller, *Biochem. Genet. 261,* 9, 1973.

11.   J. Schwarzmeir and K. Moser Verhand, *der Deutsch. Gesellsch. fur Inner. Med. 398,* 77, 1971.

12.   A.W. Murray, *Ann. Rev. Biochem. 40,* 773, 1971.

13.   T.S. Chen, U. Ishii, C. Long and H.J. Green, *J. Cell Physiol. 81,* 315, 1973.

14.   C.H.M.M. deBruyn and T.L. Oei, *Exptl. Cell Res. 450,* 79, 1973.

15.   J.J. Moore, Unpublished.

16.   H. Green and T. Chan, *Science 837,* 182, 1973.

17.   P.R. Brown and H.J. Meuwissen, Unpublished.

DISCUSSION

DR. GERALD: Howard Green told me that if you add adenosine to the cultures it is destroyed by the adenosine deaminase in the serum added to the medium.

ROCHELLE HIRSCHHORN: I know that. All I can say is that I must pass that point dealing with serum that had a low concentration of adenosine deaminase because I know that fetal calf serum has enormous amounts of the enzyme. Possibly this may explain why we need higher concentrations of adenosine to get inhibition.

ROBERT E. PARKS, JR.: The intracellular concentration of cAMP is usually in the range of 10^{-7} to 10^{-9} M and I question whether cells would encounter 1 mM concentrations of adenosine under many conditions. Perhaps you required such high concentrations of these compounds *in vitro* because they were degraded by enzymes in the serum.

DR. HADDEN: Rochelle, did you measure adenosine in any of your extracted or cultured tissues from your patients with deficiencies?

ROCHELLE HIRSCHHORN: No.

DR. HADDEN: Dr. Giblett, did the cultured fibroblasts of this patient show normal proliferation kinetics?

DR. GIBLETT: We do not yet have this information.

LAUREN PACHMAN (Children's Memorial Hospital, Chicago, Illinois): Do you have information on the ADA of fetal tissue in as much as we're using them for reconstitution?

ROCHELLE HIRSCHHORN: On amnion cells.

DR. PACHMAN: What about fetal thymus or fetal liver?

DR. PICKERING: We looked at human fetal tissue and found abundant enzyme activity in most tissues as early as 8—9 weeks gestation but we haven't looked earlier than that.

BYUNG PARK: I am interested in the possible linkage between ADA and

135

major histocompatibility complex. Dr. Meuwissen has mentioned that lymphocytes of patients with CID are poor stimulator cells in mixed leukocyte culture. That is certainly compatible with a possible defect in the expression of histocompatibility antigen on cell surface. Are there more observations of this kind and has HLA typing been done?

DR. GIBLETT: HLA typing has been done on some of the patients and, as far as I know, their HLA antigens are intact. I really don't understand the relevance of your question because you'd have to have some linkage disequilibrium in order for them to react that way.

DR. PARK: The relevance of my question is as follows: if there is linkage a deletion might conceivably occur in ADA as well as in histocompatibility complex.

DR. GIBLETT: We have considered the possibility of a deletion and abandoned it because one would have to infer that the same deletion had occurred spontaneously at least 20 times. That seems too unlikely to entertain seriously. Also, the two loci are probably not on the same chromosome.

DR. GERALD: As of June, at the Somatic Cell Hybridization and Gene Assignment Workshop, nobody could be sure whether there are one or two loci. Since then it has been decided that there is only one locus and the data suggests that it is on chromosome 20.
Somatic cell hybridization is not one that necessarily gives you an unequivocal answer. Again, this means the smallest chromosome — this is the one that is the most exchanged and therefore the one that presents the most difficulty in obtaining the kind of data which would provide a firm answer.

DR. GIBLETT: Even assuming that you're correct, I would again go back to the fact that gene mutation is a common cause of disease in many metabolic pathways. We already have more cases of ADA deficiency than we have of many other heritable metabolic defects. I don't think anyone can seriously entertain the possibility that these are due to deletions. Once you get 15 to 20 cases, the possibility of deletion is highly unlikely.

M.D. GARRICK (Beel Facility, State University of New York at Buffalo, Buffalo, New York): The argument against deletion is reasonably strong but I would like to point out that hemoglobin Lepore, which is a form of deletion, provides an example of repeated occurrence of a deletion of a particular portion of a chromosome.

DR. GIBLETT: The Lepore hemoglobins are thought to be the result of unequal crossing over.

DR. GERALD: You must realize that the anomalous crossing over is only a theory. A deletion could account for it just as well as anomalous crossing over. Don't forget the story of the Albino locus in the mouse after radiation. Many of them are deletions which involve the glucose-6-phosphatase locus. Here is an induced mutation and an example of repeatedly occurring deletion.

ROCHELLE HIRSCHHORN: Dr. Giblett has the evidence against deletion; namely, that there is some enzyme activity in the fibroblasts from these children.

SECTION IV

PYRIMIDINE STARVATION INDUCED BY ADENOSINE IN CULTURED CELLS AND ITS BEARING ON THE LYMPHOCYTE DEFICIENCY DISEASE ASSOCIATED WITH ABSENCE OF ADENOSINE DEAMINASE*

Howard Green

During the last few years, part of the work of my laboratory has been devoted to making mutant cells subject to chemical selection. Our aim was to use these mutants to construct somatic cell hybrids valuable for making chromosomal assignments for human genes.[1] For example, we developed a cell line with a mutational deficiency in the enzyme adenine phosphoribosyl transferase and a selective system in which adenine served as the sole source of AMP, making the enzyme a vital one. This enabled us to prepare a human-mouse somatic cell hybrid containing the human gene for that enzyme.[2] Subsequent work on this system by Tischfield and Ruddle[3] permitted the assignment of the human gene to chromosome No. 16. We then tried to develop an analogous selective system for adenosine kinase (AK), using adenosine as the source of cellular adenosine nucleotides.

The Effects of Exogenous Adenosine

We soon discovered that in ordinary cell culture medium, adenosine was unstable. Fig. 1 shows that this was due to the calf serum, which contains adenosine deaminase[4] in sufficient concentration to deaminate the adenosine within minutes or hours, depending on its concentration.[5] Human serum also contains appreciable deaminase but horse serum does not. It was therefore possible to test the utilization of adenosine in deaminase-free medium supplemented with horse serum.

We were surprised to find that under these conditions, adenosine in quite low concentration was toxic to the cells. At 10^{-4} to 10^{-5}M it killed the cells, and lower concentrations were inhibitory to growth (Table 1). Tests of the ability of related compounds to protect against these effects of adenosine soon showed that most pyrimidines, but not purines, when added to the culture medium, fully restored the ability of the cells to grow in the presence

---

*Aided by Grants from the National Cancer Institute.

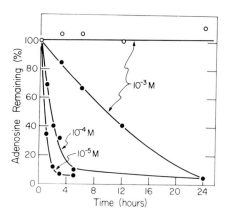

Fig. 1. Presence of adenosine deaminase in calf serum and its absence from horse serum.

○ ○ ○ horse serum, ● ● ● calf serum. (Data from Reference 5)

TABLE 1

Inhibition by Adenosine of Growth of Different Cell Lines in Medium
Free of Adenosine Deaminase

Cell Line		Lowest inhibitory adenosine concentration Moles/L (x 10^6)
Fibroblast	3T6	5
	3T6 - TM(AK⁻)	350
	3T3	2
Epithelial	HeLa	35
Lymphoid	MGL - 5	3
	L -5178y	1

of adenosine. Thus, the presence of exogenous adenosine clearly interferes with cellular pyrimidine synthesis.

When we incubated cultures for several hours in the presence of adenosine, using C^{14}-labeled aspartic acid as a tracer for pyrimidines, we found that the synthesis of labeled uridine nucleotides was much reduced and labeled orotate appeared in the medium (Fig. 2). The synthesis of UMP was evidently interrupted at this late stage of the biosynthetic pathway.

The resulting pyrimidine starvation is quickly followed by virtual emptying of the cellular pyrimidine nucleotide pool.[9,6] Fig. 3 shows the result of high pressure liquid chromatography of extracts of a human lymphoblastoid cell line, MGL-5, by the method of P. Brown.[7] Most of the ribonucleoside di- and triphosphates are readily resolved and the area under the optical density curves is proportional to the amount of nucleotide present. After 6 hours incubation in the presence of 2×10^{-5}M adenosine, the cells lost nearly all their UTP, UDP, CTP and presumptive UDPG. ATP and ADP were increased 100% and 50% respectively. The same pattern was observed in cultured fibroblasts (Fig. 4). Independent studies of the effects of exogenous adenosine and adenosine nucleotides on HeLa cells by Kaukel, Fuhrmann and Hilz[8] and Hilz and Kaukel[9] have given very similar results, both with regard to the depletion of pyrimidine nucleotides and its effects on growth.

In order to interrupt pyrimidine synthesis, the adenosine must be converted directly to AMP (Fig. 5). This is clear since 1) hypoxanthine and inosine are not lethal to cells, 2) hypoxanthine in concentration comparable to that of adenosine has little effect on the pyrimidine nucleotide pool (Fig. 4 and 3) a tubercidin-resistant subline of 3T6 possessing virtually no adenosine kinase activity (3T6-TM) is very resistant to adenosine killing (Table 1). Presumably it is the increased content of an adenosine nucleotide which reduces pyrimidine synthesis.

Interference with pyrimidine synthesis and excretion of orotate have been shown to follow the administration of 6-azauridine[10] or allopurinol.[11–13] These effects seem to be due to the nucleoside 5' phosphates. For example, the analogs 6-azauridylate[14] and 5-azaorotidylate[15] inhibit orotidylate decarboxylase competitively *in vitro*. Allopurinol ribonucleotide and XMP at concentrations of 10^{-3}M to 10^{-4}M also inhibit this enzyme very strongly,[11–13] whereas AMP is a relatively weak inhibitor.[11]

Both purine and pyrimidine synthesis require phosphoribosyl pyrophosphate (PRPP); it was shown earlier that cells exposed to orotate reduce their rate of purine synthesis[16] presumably owing to depletion of PRPP by the orotidylate phosphorylase reaction.[17] The effect of adenosine cannot be due to consumption of PRPP in the utilization of hypoxanthine produced from the adenosine since hypoxanthine does not have the

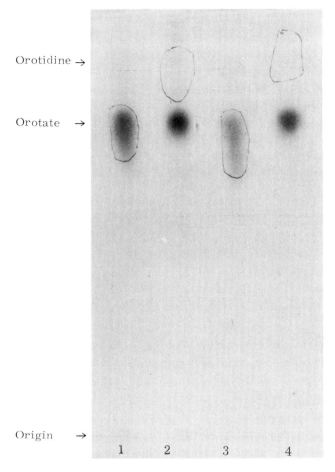

Fig. 2. Excretion of orotate into the medium by cells incubated in the presence of adenosine.

Growing cultures of 3T6 cells were incubated for three hours in medium supplemented with 10% horse serum and containing adenosine at 10^{-4}M and C^{14}-aspartate to label pyrimidines. The medium was then harvested and the proteins precipitated with perchloric acid. The pyrimidines of the supernatant were adsorbed onto charcoal, eluted with ethanol-ammonia and subjected to 2 dimensional thin layer chromatography. The most prominent radioactive spot was eluted and chromatographed in another solvent system.

The autoradiogram shows the position of the radioactive compound when co-chromatographed with unlabeled orotate (tracks 1 and 3) or unlabeled orotidine (tracks 2 and 4). Pencilled circles indicate limits of carrier orotidine. The labeled compound corresponds to orotate.[5]

145

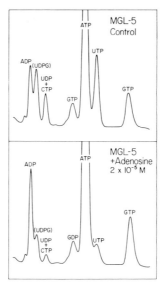

Fig. 3.   Effect of exogenous adenosine on the pyrimidine nucleotide pool of a human lymphoblastoid cell line.

High pressure liquid chromatography of perchloric acid extracts of cultures[6] shows that adenosine produces severe depletion of UTP, UDP and CTP. A peak which moves with a UDPG standard is also much reduced; this may be UDPG itself or other uridine diphosphate sugars. Analysis of smaller samples showed that ADP and ATP were increased by 50% and 100% respectively. Ordinate, O.D. 254 nm; abscissa, elution volume.

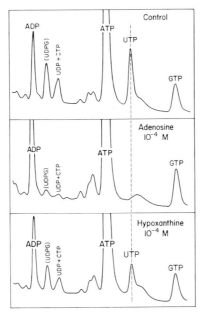

Fig. 4. Effects of adenosine and hypoxanthine on the pyrimidine nucleotide pool of 3T6 fibroblasts.

The pyrimidine nucleotide pool is greatly reduced by adenosine but very slightly affected by hypoxanthine. The identity of two of the peaks has been corrected since an earlier publication.[6]

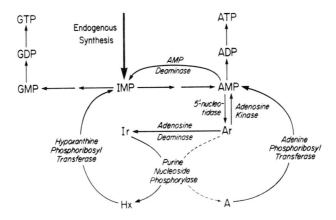

Fig. 5. The utilization of adenosine (Ar).

same effect on the cells. However, since ADP is an inhibitor of PRPP synthesis,[18,19] it seems reasonable that adenosine toxicity might be exerted through excessive regulatory reduction of the activity of PRPP synthetase. Measurement of PRPP in cells exposed to adenosine has shown a reduction in level by about 50–60%.[20] This reduction is small compared with that of the pyrimidine nucleotide pool; but it seems likely that undiminished consumption of the nucleotides by nucleic acid synthesis in the presence of even a slight choke on the synthetic pathway could result in the more profound drop in the pyrimidine nucleotide level. As shown by Krooth,[21] cells suffering from an enzyme defect in the enzymes which convert orotate to UMP have increased sensitivity to adenosine.

High concentrations of adenosine were shown earlier to produce effects on lymphocytes by Hirschhorn, Grossman and Weissmann[11] and on other cell types by numerous investigators (cited in Reference 6). We have found that at concentrations greater than 2×10^{-4}M, adenosine lethality is no longer relieved by pyrimidines, suggesting the involvement of another block. For example, Hilz and Kaukel[9] have shown that the levels of nicotinamide adenine dinucleotide in HeLa cells are reduced by high concentrations of exogenous adenosine. While the concentration of adenosine nucleotides in the tissues of animals or man might never rise sufficiently to produce this effect, they might more easily reach levels able to interfere with pyrimidine synthesis. The adenosine nucleotide concentration in mammalian cells is normally greater than 1 mM.[7]

The Role of Adenosine Deaminase

The purine scavenger pathways seem at least partly designed to help control the balance between the levels of cellular AMP and GMP. In mammalian cells the convertibility of GMP to IMP is very poor[23] but the conversion of AMP to IMP through the successive actions of 5'nucleotidase, adenosine deaminase, purine nucleoside phosphorylase and hypoxanthine phosphoribosyl transferase is very effective and may be followed by conversion of the IMP to GMP. Adenosine deaminase therefore appears to act as a regulating enzyme by reducing the level of AMP and permitting its conversion to GMP. However, if the IMP generated from adenosine is reconverted to AMP, an adenosine cycle is created. It was predicted[23] and found[24] that the unrestrained operation of this cycle would lead to loss of purines from the cell. It must therefore be the role of adenosine kinase to oppose the action of adenosine deaminase by lowering the adenosine concentration.

When 3T6 cells were exposed to tracer amounts of tritiated adenosine, both the guanosine nucleotides and adenosine nucleotides were labeled. It could be estimated that of the labeled adenosine metabolized, about 20% was deaminated and the rest converted directly to AMP. This is in good agreement with the results of earlier studies of Ehrlich ascites tumor cells by Snyder and Henderson.[25] At higher adenosine concentrations, a greater proportion of the adenosine is deaminated.[25]

The adenosine deaminase of most cell types is probably adequate to deal with endogenously generated adenosine but not with exogenous adenosine. When added to cultures of fibroblast or lymphoblastoid cells, adenosine forces a rise in internal levels of the adenosine nucleotides, in spite of the presence of the cellular deaminase (Fig. 3). Some cell types may be specially equipped to deal with exogenous adenosine; for example, the deaminase is extremely active in intestinal epithelium,[26] perhaps because this rapidly growing cell type would otherwise be affected by adenosine absorbed from dietary nucleic acid, or because it is necessary to prevent the entrance of the absorbed adenosine into the blood. Since the spleen (and usually the lymph nodes) contain high levels of the enzyme,[26] they may also require an unusual amount of protection from adenosine.

Another possible route for the elimination of adenosine nucleotides is by deamination of AMP to give IMP. This reaction has been most studied in extracts of muscle.[27] In other cell types it may be less important.[28] In experiments on fibroblasts incubated with tracer amounts of labeled adenine, we found that within an hour the ADP and ATP were well labeled; but as no label appeared in GDP and GTP, there was no demonstrable deamination of AMP. Nevertheless, in the presence of aminopterin, adenine can serve as the sole purine source for fibroblasts lacking the enzyme hypoxanthine phosphoribosyl transferase,[23] so it seems that at least under purine starvation conditions, AMP deaminase can function sufficiently to provide GMP from AMP. Deamination of adenosine is probably the principal means by which cells reduce their concentration of adenosine nucleotides but in some cells the AMP deaminase may be an adequate alternate route. This might explain why only certain cell types seem to be affected by absence of adenosine deaminase.

A possible test of the importance of adenosine deaminase in wild type cells would be to treat the cells with inhibitors of this enzyme. If adenosine deaminase is the principal enzyme eliminating adenosine nucleotides, coformycin, a very effective inhibitor,[25] should produce an increase in the adenosine nucleotide pool and possibly a toxic effect similar to that of exogenous adenosine.

Until recently there was thought to be no adenosine phosphorylase in mammalian cells. By the use of more sensitive methods, it has been found that purine nucleoside phosphorylase will use adenosine or adenine as substrate, though with very low efficiency.[29,25] Since any adenine formed in this way from adenosine would likely be reconverted to AMP by the phosphoribosyl transferase, no loss of adenosine nucleotides would result. Adenine produced from adenosine might be eliminated from the cell by excretion but in studies of labeled purine excretion from cultured cells, we were unable to find adenine in the medium.

Possible Consequences of Absence of Adenosine Deaminase

This line of reasoning suggests that absence of adenosine deaminase could impair the regulation of the adenosine nucleotides in some cell types, leading to accumulation of these nucleotides and interference with pyrimidine synthesis. An increase in cellular adenosine nucleotides could originate (a) from endogenously generated adenosine nucleotides and adenosine and (b) from adenosine arising exogenously from any source, such as dietary nucleic acids or cell death and breakdown. If adenosine deaminase were absent from intestinal mucosa and from serum, there would be no barrier to the transport of absorbed adenosine to all cells and the adenosine should be detectable in the serum.

In either case, the affected cells may be killed or their growth prevented, depending on the degree of pyrimidine starvation. The effect should be more severe for rapidly growing cell types with a large pyrimidine requirement. If the cell type involved were not killed but only inhibited in nucleic acid accumulation and growth, it might be restored to activity by providing a pyrimidine source. This possibility should be examined for the disease which is the subject of this meeting.

Pyrimidine Sources for Mammalian Cells

When endogenous pyrimidine synthesis is prevented by exogenous adenosine a number of pyrimidines can be utilized by the cell (Table 2) but not with equal effectiveness. Their routes of utilization are shown in Fig. 5. Uridine is the most directly utilized; uridine kinase converts it to UMP. CTP is made from UTP.[30,31] Both triphosphates are then available for nucleic acid synthesis. Uridine is effective at 10^{-5}M or less in cell cultures whose endogenous synthesis is blocked by adenosine.

All other pyrimidine sources also require uridine kinase for their utilization. This is clear from Fig. 6, for cytidine kinase and uridine kinase are the same enzyme.[32] Absence of uridine kinase in a cell makes it unable to utilize any pyrimidine source for survival in the presence of adenosine.[33]

The efficiency with which the different pyrimidines can serve as source probably depends on the number of reactions necessary for their utilization. For example, uracil utilization depends not only on uridine kinase but also on

150

TABLE 2

Ability of Pyrimidines to Support Growth of 3T6 Cells in the
Presence of Adenosine (0.1 mM)

I Growth	II No Growth
Uridine	Cytosine
Uracil	Orotidine
Cytidine	Orotate
Deoxyuridine	Thymidine
Deoxycytidine	——
	Hypoxanthine
	Inosine
	Guanine
	Guanosine
	Deoxyguanosine

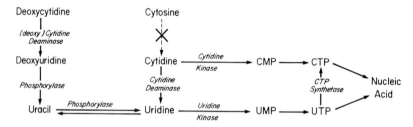

Fig. 6. Pyrimidine sources for cells whose endogenous synthesis is blocked by adenosine.

Cytidine kinase = uridine kinase.[32]

Deoxycytidine deaminase = cytidine deaminase.[35]

phosphorylase to generate uridine. Probably for this reason it must be present in somewhat higher concentrations than uridine in order to support growth. Cytidine, if it is to supply uridine nucleotides as well as cytidine nucleotides, must be deaminated by cytidine deaminase. It is less effective as the sole pyrimidine source than uridine. Deoxyuridine utilization requires still a fourth reaction. These nucleosides must be present in even higher concentrations than uracil or cytidine in order to support growth in the presence of adenosine. Neither cytosine nor thymidine is effective at any concentration, as they cannot be converted to ribonucleosides in mammalian cells. Possibly the most efficient pyrimidine source would be a balanced combination of uridine and cytidine, for no conversion of one base to the other would then be necessary.

An anology can be drawn between the two genetic defects, orotic aciduria and absence of adenosine deaminase, since an impairment in pyrimidine synthesis accompanied by excretion of orotic acid has been demonstrated in one and, on the basis of the cell culture model, is likely to occur in the other. Before the existence of the disease associated with absence of adenosine deaminase was brought to our attention by Dr. Cedric Long, we suggested,[5] that orotic aciduria might result from a defect in adenosine metabolism as well as through mutation in the enzymes converting orotate to UMP.[21] On the other hand, if absence of adenosine deaminase affects the level of adenosine nucleotides in only a few cell types, the excretion of orotate might not be appreciable at the level of the whole organism.

Pyrimidine starvation from any cause would be expected to affect the hematopoietic and lymphoid systems, since some cells of these systems are among the most rapidly growing cell types. As a provision of an exogenous source of uridine has been successful in the treatment or orotic aciduria,[34] it seems reasonable that it should alleviate the effects of absence of adenosine deaminase, if the stem cell population has not been destroyed.

REFERENCES

1.   H. Green, Wistar Institute Symposium Monograph No. 9, V. Defendi (Ed.), Wistar Institute Press, p. 51, 1969.

2.   T. Kusano, C. Long and H. Green, *Proc. Nat. Acad. Sci. 68,* 82, 1971.

3.   J.A. Tischfield and F.H. Riddle, *Proc. Nat. Acad. Sci.,* (in press).

4.   J.C. Cory, G. Weinbaum and R.J. Suhadolnik, *Arch. Biochem. Biophys. 118,* 418, 1967.

5. K. Ishii and H. Green, *J. Cell Sci. 13,* 429, 1973.

6. H. Green and T.-s. Chan, *Science 182,* 836, 1973.

7. P.R. Brown, *J. Chromatog. 52,* 257, 1970.

8. E. Kaukel, U. Fuhrmann and H. Hilz, *Biochem. Biophys. Res. Commun. 48,* 1516, 1972.

9. H. Hilz and E. Kaukel, *Mol. & Cell Biochem. 1,* 229, 1973.

10. S.S. Cardoso, P. Calabresi and R.E. Handschumacher, *Canc. Res. 21,* 1551, 1961.

11. W.N. Kelley and T.D. Beardmore, *Science 169,* 388, 1970.

12. R.M. Fox, D. Royse-Smith and W.J. O'Sullivan, *Science 168,* 861, 1970.

13. W.N. Kelley, T.D. Beardmore, I.H. Fox and J.C. Meade, *Biochem. Pharmacol. 20,* 1471, 1971.

14. R.E. Handschumacher, *J. Biol. Chem. 235,* 2917, 1970.

15. A. Čihák and F. Šorm, *Biochim. Biophys. Acta 149,* 314, 1967.

16. S. Rajalakshmi and R.E. Handschumacher, *Biochim. Biophys. Acta 155,* 317, 1968.

17. W.N. Kelley, I.H. Fox and J.B. Wyngaarden, *Biochim. Biophys. Acta 215,* 512, 1970.

18. P.C.L. Wong and A.W. Murray, *Biochemistry 8,* 1608, 1969.

19. A. Hershko, E. Razin and J. Mager, *Biochim. Biophys. Acta 184,* 64, 1969.

20. M. Meuth and H. Green (in preparation).

21. R.S. Krooth, *Cold Spring Harbor Symposium Quant. Biol. 29,* 189, 1964.

22. R. Hirschhorn, J. Grossman and G. Weissmann, *Proc. Soc. Exptl. Biol. Med. 133,* 1361, 1970.

23. H. Green and K. Ishii, *J. Cell. Sci. 11,* 173, 1972.

24. T.-s. Chan, K. Ishii, C. Long and H. Green, *J. Cell Physiol. 81,* 315,

1973.

25. F.F. Snyder and J.F. Henderson, *J. Biol. Chem. 248,* 5899, 1973.

26. T.G. Brady and C.I. O'Donovan, *Comp. Biochem. Physiol. 14,* 101, 1965.

27. J. Lowenstein and K. Tornheim, *Science 171,* 397, 1971.

28. A.W. Murray, D.C. Elliott and M.R. Atkinson, *in* Progress in Nucleic Acid Research and Molecular Biology, Vol. 10, J.N. Davidson and W.E. Cohn (Eds.), p. 87, 1970.

29. T.P. Zimmerman, N.B. Gersten, A.F. Ross and R.P. Miech, *Canad. J. Biochem. 49,* 1050, 1971.

30. C.W. Long and A.B. Pardee, *J. Biol. Chem. 242,* 4715, 1967.

31. C.R. Savage and H. Weinfield, *J. Biol. Chem. 245,* 2529, 1970.

32. A. Orengo, *J. Biol. Chem. 244,* 2204, 1969.

33. L. Medrano and H. Green, *Cell 1,* 23, 1974.

34. L.H. Smith, C.M. Huguley and J.A. Bain, *in* Metabolic Basis of Inherited Disease, J.B. Stanbury, J.B. Wyngaarden and D.S. Fredrickson (Eds.), 3rd edition, McGraw-Hill, p. 1003, 1972.

ISOPRINOSINE, A PURINE DERIVATIVE; METABOLIC, IMMUNOLOGICAL AND ANTIVIRAL EFFECTS

A.J. Glasky
E.H. Pfadenhauer
R. Settineri
T. Ginsberg

The search for effective and safe antiviral agents has been relatively unproductive due to the fact that the intracellular biochemical systems required for viral replication parallel those involved in normal essential metabolic functions of the host.[1,2] The major approaches to combating viral infections can be classified in two categories: (1) chemical impairment of the etiological agent or its replication; i.e., the antimetabolites and (2) enhancement of host defense mechanism; i.e., interferon and immunological response.

Antimetabolites, such as IUDR, N-methylisatin-B-thiosemicarbazone and amantadine, have low to moderate levels of efficacy, narrow spectrum of activity, short duration of protection and are high in toxicity.

Interferon itself has proven impractical and attention has been directed toward interferon inducers. The inducers show broader spectrum of activity in animals than the antimetabolites but undesirable features such as toxicity, antigenicity and, in particular, a lack of efficacy in natural infections in man.

The immunological approach is not universally applicable because of the impracticability of vaccinating against every virus strain or mutant and the uncertainty regarding the cumulative effects of repeated administration of antigenically foreign materials. However, the fact remains that the immunological approach has been the only one that has proven to be effective in control of viral disease.

Potentially effective chemical agents which enhance host cell response may have been deemed failures because they did not obey the classical dogma: Antiviral = kill virus. A new substance[3] which appears to offer a somewhat novel approach to antiviral therapy is Isoprinosine (T.M. Newport Pharmaceuticals International, Inc., Newport Beach, California).

Isoprinosine (generic name, Inosiplex, whose structure is seen in Figure 1) is a complex of 1 mole of inosine and 3 moles of p-acetamidobenzoate salt of

Figure 1 →

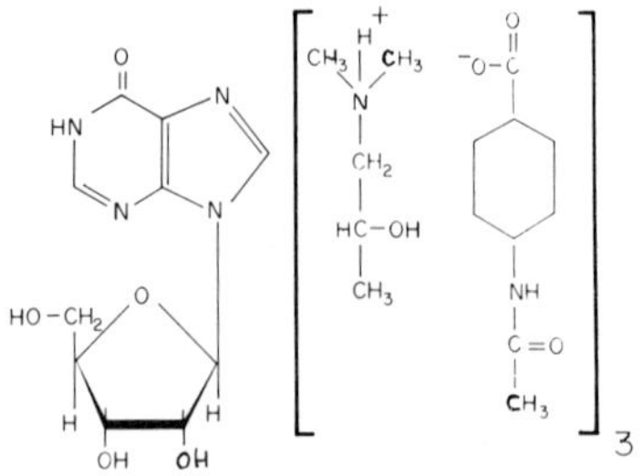

ISOPRINOSINE®

TABLE 1

Antiviral Effect of Isoprinosine in Tissue Culture

Virus Strain	Tissue	Reference
Influenza A_2 Bethesda	PMK	Muldoon, Menzy, Jackson[6]
Influenza A_2 Hong Kong	PMK	Muldoon, Menzy, Jackson[6]
		Ginsberg, Settineri, Pfadenhauer and Glasky[7]
Influenza B Maryland	PMK	Muldoon, Menzy, Jackson[6]
Influenza B Massachusetts	PMK	Muldoon, Menzy, Jackson[6]
Herpes Hominis	WI-38	Muldoon, Menzy, Jackson[6]
Herpes Hominis Type 2	Human Amnion	Chang, Weinstein[8]
Herpes Hominis LU	PRK	Gordon, Brown[9]
Rhino 44	HeLa	Ginsberg, Settineri, Pfadenhauer and Glasky[7]
Vaccinia	Human Amnion	Chang, Weinstein[8]
Eastern Equine Encephalitis	Chick Fibroblast	Chang, Weinstein[8]

1-dimethylamino-2-propanol. This substance has been shown to be non-toxic in a variety of species including man.[4] To date, we have not seen any untoward reactions after acute or chronic administration to man except for temporary elevations in uric acid, which is the end product of the metabolism of the purine portion of the drug.[5]

Isoprinosine has been shown (Table 1) to be active against a variety of viruses in tissue culture[6,9] when certain factors are taken into consideration in the design of the experiments. Since the drug is rapidly metabolized, it must be administered in adequate doses, replenished frequently and maintained for sufficient duration.[7] The challenge dose of virus is also critical.[6] Isoprinosine appears to be more active therapeutically than prophylactically and does not induce interferon.[10]

Isoprinosine has been shown (Table 2) to be active against both RNA and DNA viruses in animals.[6,8,10,11,12] Similarly, challenge dose of virus, adequacy of drug dosage including amount given, duration and timing of onset of therapy are critical factors that must be taken into consideration in order to demonstrate antiviral effects.

While the studies shown in Tables 1 and 2 were successful in demonstrating antiviral activity of Isoprinosine, a number of published reports have appeared in which activity was not demonstrable due to lack of consideration of the aforementioned critical parameters.[10,13] Notwithstanding this more apparent than real controversy regarding the tissue culture and animal efficacy of Isoprinosine, the clinical studies in man directed toward therapeutic treatment of naturally occurring viral infections have been astonishingly successful.

Table 3 represents a compilation of the results of a number of published clinical studies.[14—37] Relief occurs within 24-48 hours in the following acute symptoms when present:
1. Fever, although Isoprinosine has no direct antipyretic action;
2. Pain, although Isoprinosine has no direct analgesic action;
3. Nasal and respiratory congestion, although Isoprinosine has no direct antihistamine or anti-inflammatory action.

The erythemas also show rapid resolution.

In vivo and *in vitro* studies on the mechanism of action of Isoprinosine have shown that it is neither a metabolic inhibitor nor an interferon inducer. Studies showing its ability to stimulate certain aspects of protein synthesis led us to consider the hypothesis that its activity might involve the immune system.

Studies were designed to evaluate the interaction of Isoprinosine with elements of the immune response. Having demonstrated that Influenza A_2 is sensitive to the action of Isoprinosine in the mouse, we chose this model to investigate effects of immunosuppression on the therapeutic action of

TABLE 2

Antiviral Effect of Isoprinosine in Animals

Virus Strain	Animal	Reference
Influenza A Bethesda	Mice	Muldoon, Menzy, Jackson[6]
Influenza	Mice	Chang, Weinstein[8]
Influenza A_2	Mice	Glasky, Settineri, Lynes [11]
Influenza A_2	Mice	Gordon, Brown[12]
Influenza PR8	Mice	Gordon, Brown [12]
Herpes Hominis Type 2	Hamster	Chang, Weinstein[8]
Herpes	Hamster	Gordon, Brown[12]
Fibroma	Rabbit	Glasgow, Galasso[10]

TABLE 3

Therapeutic Use of Isoprinosine in Naturally Occurring
Infections

Disease	Number of Patients Treated	Reference
Bronchiolitis	99	14,15,16,17,18
Chicken Pox	142	15,16,17,18,19,20, 21,22,23,24,25,26
Hemorrhagic Fever (Juni)	18	27
Hepatitis (HAA-)	147	15,17,18,19,21,25, 28,29,30,31
Herpes Simplex	221	15,17,18,21,23,24, 26,32,33,34,35
Herpes Zoster	69	18,21,22,24,25,32, 33,34,35
Influenza	299	15,16,17,18,23,24, 36
Measles	186	17,18,19,20,23,25, 26,34
Mumps	59	15,18,21,23,24
Rhinopharyngitis	104	15,17,18,24,37
Rubella	20	21

Isoprinosine.[38]

Isoprinosine or saline was administered orally 24 hours following intranasal instillation of the virus. Cortisone acetate was given subcutaneously once daily for 14 days, with or without Isoprinosine. To analyze the data, cumulative proportions of dead animals were transformed to probit values. Linear regression analyses were performed on these values and the results are represented in Figure 2.

Cortisone alone was shown to enhance the death rate significantly, compared with controls. The Isoprinosine-treated group has a significantly lower death rate. The two compounds given together resulted in a fatality rate which was significantly greater than the control value but not significantly different from the cortisone alone.

Since it was reasoned that another way of producing a similar reduction of circulating lymphocytes would be the administration of antilymphocyte serum (ALS), an analogous experiment was set up using a single injection of rabbit anti-mouse lymphocyte serum in place of cortisone treatment.

The results showed that ALS-treated animals have a faster death rate than the saline controls while Isoprinosine alone gave a lower death rate. The combined treatment was not different from ALS alone and significantly reduced the protective effect of Isoprinosine.

Both cortisone and ALS enhanced the progress of infection and death, whereas Isoprinosine retarded it. When Isoprinosine was used in combination with either immunosuppressive agent, its therapeutic effect was obliterated.

The animal data are consistent with the hypothesis that the action of Isoprinosine is dependent upon an intact immune system and that its antiviral action may in part be due to facilitation of some facet of the immune response.

Three independent double-blind clinical studies[36,39,40] in man have been carried out using the prophylactic administration of Isoprinosine to subjects who received a live virus challenge. The design of these studies preceded our awareness of the greater activity of Isoprinosine in therapeutic rather than prophylactic type of experimental protocol. However, production of antibody (AB) was measured in these studies and an evaluation of the immune enhancement hypothesis was undertaken.

Longley, Dunning and Waldman[36] administered Isoprinosine (2.5g. b.i.d.) or placebo to groups of 15 subjects 2 days prior to and daily for 10 days following intranasal instillation of Influenza A_2 Hong Kong virus. The geometric mean rise in serum neutralizing AB titers was 14-fold for the placebo group and 24-fold for the drug group. This difference, although not statistically significant, may suggest a drug effect on AB formation. Virus isolation conducted over the 4-day period beginning 8 hours post-challenge showed a significantly lower number of positive isolations in the drug-treated

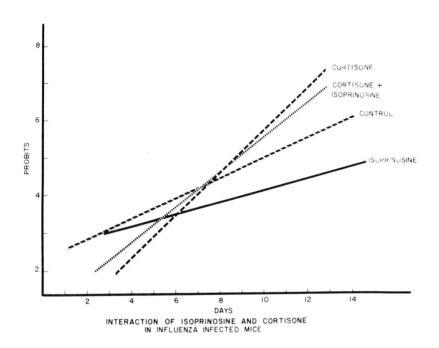

Figure 2

group (p = 0.05). Thus, the apparent AB increase is not explainable on the basis of increased amount of virus present since the virus shedding data contradict this.

A mixed rhinovirus (RV9 and RV31) challenge was employed in a double-blind study with human volunteers by Soto *et al.*,[39] who administered Isoprinosine (1.5g. q.i.d.) 2 days before and daily for 7 days following concurrent intranasal inoculation with both strains of rhinovirus. The placebo and drug groups consisted of 22 and 23 subjects respectively. Nasal washings were collected for viral isolation and blood was sampled for serum neutralizing AB. Subjects with appreciable initial AB titer were not eliminated from the study by the investigators. Either isolation of virus, or a 4-fold or greater increase in specific AB titer, or both, was taken as a criterion for diagnosing infection with the particular strain of virus.

In Figure 3, the changes in geometric mean AB titer from pre-drug to day 17 were plotted vs. diagnosed infection. The categories shown are:

1. Diagnosed as RV9 only;
2. Diagnosed as RV31 only;
3. Diagnosed as RV9 and RV31;
4. Uninfected.

The antibody measured in each category is also shown.

Striking differences in AB elevations between the drug and placebo treated subjects were evident in the RV31-only infection (second set) and the mixed infection when measuring AB change for RV9 (p $<$ 0.006). No difference between drug and placebo AB changes were observed in other groups.

It appears from these results that there is a difference in AB response to the two rhinovirus strains, the RV9 strain being somewhat more antigenic, since a large rise in AB was noted in the placebo group. The drug appears to enhance AB response against RV31 in singly infected subjects who do not show an AB response when placebo was administered. Singly infected RV9 subjects which responded with AB formation under placebo conditions did not respond to the drug.

In the mixed infection group, the AB responsiveness to RV9 was suppressed by the presence of the other viruses under placebo conditions. This lack of AB responsiveness was overcome by drug treatment.

Apparently under those conditions in which host antibody response is substantial (either based on the antigenicity of the virus or the immuno-competence of the host) the drug does not seem to produce an enhancement of AB production. However, under those circumstances in which an adequate response is not achieved, Isoprinosine seems to enhance the production of AB. Under the conditions of mixed infections, other factors may be involved.

While the data in humans is still somewhat preliminary, a drug induced

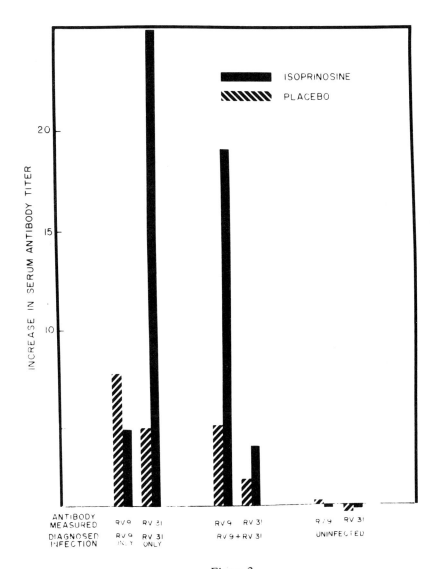

Figure 3

increase in AB production has been seen. The basis for the variability between different strains of viruses are yet to be explained and additional studies in these antiviral infection models are in progress.

Considering the fact that Isoprinosine has the natural purine inosine as one of its components and the possibility that Isoprinosine may exert its antiviral activity possibly in part due to an immunostimulant mechanism, it was natural for us to turn our interest to the immunodeficient state that was characterized by a defect in purine metabolism, combined immunodeficiency with an ADA defect.

Studying the metabolism of Isoprinosine in normal healthy adults had led our laboratory to the development of rapid, sensitive, analytical techniques, particularly the use of high pressure liquid chromatography for the separation of purine bases, nucleosides and nucleotides. The methods for analysis of nucleotides are essentially those previously reported by Brown.[40] Nucleosides and bases are analyzed using a new method recently published[41] from our laboratory employing silicic acid and an organic solvent system in the Varian LCA-4100 High Pressure Liquid Chromatography System. The advantages of the new methodology are that they allow us to analyze samples of as little as 250 microliters of whole blood and achieve separation and quantitation of the main components in approximately 30 minutes. The identity of the different components and the various peaks is confirmed by enzymatic methods. Overlapping nucleosides and bases can be determined by shifts in the peaks produced by enzymatic reaction.

This methodology has been applied to the analysis of blood samples from three patients. These samples were kindly supplied by Dr. Richard Pickering of Dalhousie University. Two hospitalized children (L.S. and S.S.) served as controls for an immunodeficient child (A.M.) having an adenosine deaminase (ADA) defect. In the ADA deficient patient, the production of inosine from adenosine is impaired, thus we are particularly interested in noting the clinical effects of the administration of Isoprinosine, a biologically utilizable form of inosine, to this type of patient. We are particularly aware of the limited number of subjects in this study but because of the interesting nature of the results obtained we felt it would be worthwhile to report these preliminary results to this group. We hope to extend the analysis to a larger number of subjects.

Table 4 shows the level of purine metabolites in plasma from the two control patients and the ADA deficient patient. In this table the designation "ud" indicates that we were unable to detect measurable amounts of the particular compound. The lower limit is indicated in the average column by a value and an asterisk and does not represent actual determinations.

Focusing our attention first on the pre-drug levels as compared to controls,

TABLE 4

Purine Metabolite Levels in Plasma
(μg/ml)

	Control Patients			Immunodeficient Patients	
	L.F.	S. S.	Average	A.M.	
				Pre Drug	Post Drug
ADO	ud	ud	< 0.60*	ud	ud
ADE	ud	ud	< 0.40*	ud	ud
GUO	ud	ud	< 0.60*	ud	ud
GUA	ud	ud	< 0.40*	ud	ud
INO	1.48	1.90	1.69	0.99	1.29
HX	3.91	3.13	3.52	0.74	1.07
XAO	na	na	na	na	na
XAN	0.51	0.43	0.47	0.52	0.89
UA	32.1	41.7	36.9	9.6	17.1

*   Approximate limit of detectability

ud = undetectable

na = not analyzed

167

we note the depressed levels of inosine, hypoxanthine and uric acid while the level of xanthine was normal. We were not able to find any detectable level of adenine or adenosine in plasma.

The ADA deficient patient was given 100 mg/kilo of Isoprinosine orally and a blood sample obtained one hour after drug administration. The values obtained are indicated in the last column. We see an increase in most of the measurable purine metabolites, however, only xanthine increased to a level which exceeded that of the control patients. There was no appearance of any new purine metabolites after drug treatment that were not present prior to drug treatment.

Table 5 reports the analyses of purine metabolites in TCA soluble extracts of erythrocytes. Again, first comparing the pre-drug samples from the ADA deficient patient with the controls, we notice that the total adenine nucleotide level was lower. We have not attributed a great deal of significance to the differences in levels of the individual nucleotides because of the possibility of interconversions. We were not able to detect adenine or adenosine in the control patients but a significant level of adenine was determined in the ADA deficient patient. The guanine nucleotides were not present in sufficient quantities to detect any differences using our methodology. IMP values appeared normal; however, hypoxanthine was low. The one-hour post-drug sample showed an elevation in the total adenine nucleotides, the increase of which seemed to be primarily due to elevation of ATP. Both IMP and hypoxanthine levels increased; however, there was no detectable increase in the inosine levels in RBC under conditions when the plasma did show an increase in inosine. Even after drug treatment the guanine nucleotides were in too low a concentration to show any changes.

Thus, the ADA deficient disease has been metabolically characterized most noticeably by the presence of substantial quantities of adenine in the RBC but not in plasma. Adenosine was not found in either RBC or plasma.

Total adenine nucleotide levels, as well as hypoxanthine and uric acid were markedly lower in the ADA patient.

Administration of Isoprinosine brought the adenine nucleotide levels up to normal, without a concomitant rise in adenosine or adenine levels. Also elevated after drug were IMP and hypoxanthine in RBC's and inosine, hypoxanthine, xanthine and uric acid in plasma.

SUMMARY

Applying newly developed methodology, we have partially characterized the metabolic profile of an immunodeficient patient with an adenosine deaminase defect. We showed the presence of abnormal quantities of

TABLE 5

Purine Metabolite Levels in Erythrocyte
(mM/L Packed RBC)

	Control Patients			Immunodeficient Patients	
	L. F.	S. S.	Average	A.M.	
				Pre Drug	Post Drug
ATP	0.51	0.56	0.54	0.41	0.93
ADP	0.32	0.36	0.34	0.25	0.31
AMP	0.34	0.44	0.39	0.15	0.12
Total A-Nucleotide	1.17	1.36	1.26	0.81	1.36
ADO	ud	ud	<0.01*	ud	ud
ADE	ud	ud	<0.01*	0.05	0.05
GDP	0.01	0.01	0.01	tr	tr
GMP	0.02	0.03	0.02	0.03	0.03
GUO	ud	ud	<0.01*	ud	ud
GUA	ud	ud	<0.01*	ud	ud
IMP	0.05	0.14	0.10	0.08	0.19
INO	ud	ud	<0.01*	ud	ud
HX	0.06	0.07	0.06	0.02	0.09
XAO	ud	ud	<0.01*	ud	ud
XAN	ud	ud	0.01*	ud	ud

* Approximate limit of detectability

tr = trace

ud = undetectable

adenine and a deficiency of adenine nucleotides in erythrocytes, as well as a deficiency in plasma inosine and oxypurines, particularly uric acid. Isoprinosine, a source of biologically utilizable inosine, was administered to the patient and a tendency to restore normal levels of the purine metabolic intermediates was observed.

The increased levels of adenine nucleotides caused by administration of Isoprinosine to the adenosine deaminase deficient patient may be important due to the known roles of cyclic AMP and cyclic GMP in the regulation of certain aspects of the immune response.[42] The absence of improvement in the clinical picture, even though there was a partial restoration of a normal purine metabolic profile, might be explained by one of the following: (1) the patient was not on Isoprinosine for sufficient duration to affect clinical improvement, (2) the increase in adenine nucleotides might have had a deleterious effect on the immune system or (3) the metabolic profile and the adenosine deaminase defect may not be directly related to the immunodeficiency.

In conclusion, we have presented data showing: (1) the effect of Isoprinosine as an antiviral agent acting at least in part by enhancement of certain facets of the immune response and (2) the ability of Isoprinosine to partially restore the normal purine metabolic profile in a combined immunodeficient patient with an adenosine deaminase defect.

REFERENCES

1. L. Weinstein and T.W. Chang, *N. Engl. J. Med. 289,* 725, 1973.

2. M.R. Hilleman, *in* Immunity in Viral and Rickettsial Diseases, A. Kohn and M.A. Klingberg (Eds.), p. 167, Plenum Press, New York, 1972.

3. E.R. Brown and P. Gordon, *Fed. Proc. 29,* 684, 1970.

4. T.E. Lynes, *The Pharmacologist 12,* 271,1970.

5. C. Fareed and H.R. Tyler, *Neurology 21,* 937, 1971.

6. R.L. Muldoon, L. Menzy and G.G. Jackson, *Antimicrob. Agents Chemother. 2,* 224, 1972.

7. T. Ginsberg, R. Settineri, E. Pfadenhauer and A.J. Glasky, *Abstr. Amer. Soc. Microbiol.,* p. 206, 1973.

8. T.W. Chang and L. Weinstein, *Amer. J. Med. Sci. 265,* 143, 1972.

9. P. Gordon and E.R. Brown, *Fed. Proc. 32,* 703, 1973.

10. L.A. Glasgow and G.J. Galasso, *J. Infect. Dis.126,* 162, 1972.

11. A.J. Glasky, R. Settineri and T.E. Lynes, *Proc. VIIth Int. Congress Chemother. 1,* A-5/19, 1971.

12. P. Gordon and E.R. Brown, *Can. J. Microbiol. 18,* 1463, 1972.

13. H.J. Eggers, A. Neufahrt and H. Rolly, *Deut. Med. Wochenschr. 97,* 1156, 1972.

14. G. Antonini *et al., Jornada Med. (Argent.) 343,* 4, 1971.

15. A.L. Cohen *et al., Prensa Med. Argent. 60,* 267, 1973.

16. J. Ink and G.M. Antonini, *Prensa Univer. (Argent.) 324,* 6121, 1970.

17. J. Ink *et al., Prensa Med. Argent. 57,* 2050, 1971.

18. J. Ink *et al., Prensa Med. Argent. 58,* 1875, 1971.

19. J.L. deLune Solano and J.dC. Silva Baeza, *El Medico (Mex.) 23,* 57, 1973.

20. C.G. Lara *et al., Med. J. Guatemala Soc. Sec. Inst. 2,* 2, 1972.

21. A. Minarro *et al., Sem. Med. (Argent.) 80,* 362, 1973.

22. B. Nudenberg *et al., Orientacion Med. (Argent.) 21,* 846, 1972.

23. B. Nunan and E. Tonelli, *J. Pediatr. (Brazil) 37,* 325, 1972.

24. M.E. Pacheco, *Rev. Med. Costa Rica 40,* 27, 1973.

25. M.A. Salas *et al., Orientacion Med. (Argent.) 21,* 551, 1972.

26. C. Stefano *et al., Orientacion Med. (Argent.) 20,* 342, 1971.

27. J. Ink *et al., Prensa Med. Argent. 59,* 542, 1972.

28. E.A. Dainko, *in* Abstr. XIth Intersci. Conf. Antimicrob. Agents Chemother., p. 30, 1971.

29. J. Ink *et al., Jornada Med. (Argent.) 349,* 6, 1971.

30. R.L. Jao *et al., J. Manila Med. Soc. 10,* 93, 1972.

31. M. Roncoroni, *Orientacion Med. (Argent.) 79,* 995, 1972.

32. M.P. Ahumada, D. Amezquita and C.E. Biro, *El Medico (Mex.)* 5, 78, 1972.

33. G. Marcone *et al.*, *Sem Med. (Argent.)* 79, 995, 1972.

34. J.C. Muracciole, J.S. Vilarino and M.A. Muracciole, *Rev. Circ. Argent. Odontol.* 35, 22, 1972.

35. T.H. Steinberg and E. Macotela Ruiz, *Prensa Med. Mex.* 37, 159, 1972.

36. S. Longley, R.L. Dunning and R.H. Waldman, *Antimicrob. Agents Chemother.* 3, 506, 1973.

37. B.M. Limson, *Philipp. J. Microbiol. Infect. Dis.* 1, 36, 1972.

38. T.E. Lynes, M. Anderson and R.A. Settineri, *in* Abstr. XIIth Intersci. Conf. Antimicrob. Agents Chemother., p. 48, 1972.

39. A.J. Soto, T.S. Hall and S.E. Reed, *Antimicrob. Agents Chemother.* 3, 332, 1973.

40. P.R. Brown, High Pressure Liquid Chromatography, Academic Press, New York, 1973.

CYCLIC NUCLEOTIDES AND LYMPHOCYTE METABOLISM, FUNCTION AND DEVELOPMENT

John W. Hadden*

Since Earl Sutherland's original formulation of the role played by cyclic 3' 5' adenosine monophosphate (cyclic AMP) as an intracellular mediator of epinephrine and glucagon action, the concept has emerged that a variety of hormones and hormone-like substances interact with receptors at the cell surface to produce an increase in the intracellular level of cyclic AMP through an increase in the activity of membrane-bound adenylate cyclase. Cyclic AMP then modulates the activity of a variety of intracellular enzyme processes, possibly by activating one or more protein kinases. This second messenger system has been demonstrated to be present in virtually every nucleated cell in the body and to subserve the modulation of a number of differentiated processes within these cells.

Recent evidence[1,2-8] indicates that the cellular levels of the other naturally occurring cyclic nucleotide and cyclic 3' 5' guanosine monophosphate (cyclic GMP) are similarly increased by hormones and hormone-like substances many of which are thought to act at the cell surface. The hormonal agents shown to increase cyclic GMP levels are those which either do not affect cyclic AMP levels (e.g., acetylcholine, serotonin, oxytocin, prostaglandin F_2a), or reputedly lower them (e.g., insulin and norepinephrine).

The physiologic and metabolic responses stimulated by hormonal agents acting on one or the other of the two cyclic nucleotide systems are generally distinct in such a way that suggest the two systems operate in an antagonistic yet complementary manner in regulating biological events. This concept forms the basis of the Yin Yang Hypothesis of biological control advanced by Goldberg, Hadden et al.[2,6-8]

Among the initial observations upon which this hypothesis was based were certain observations made in the lymphocyte which served to relate cyclic GMP and cyclic AMP to the process of cellular proliferation.[6] A number of previous observations have supported the concept that cyclic AMP plays an

---

*Established Investigator of the American Heart Association.

antiproliferative role and acts to promote differentiation and differentiated function. Observations to be described herein serve to support this concept in its application to the lymphocyte and to present evidence to support the complementary view that cyclic GMP is related to both the modulation and induction of lymphocyte proliferation and to certain differentiated functions presumed to be related to proliferation in the lymphocyte.

The studies reviewed in this manuscript concerning the role of both cyclic nucleotides in the biology of the lymphocyte are virtually all *in vitro* studies in which the metabolism and function of isolated lymphocytes have been studied using single hormonal agents often in combination with agents which simulate the action of antigen. Virtually all of these studies concern the thymocyte and thymus-dependent ("T") lymphocyte as, unfortunately, little information exists concerning the antibody producing ("B") lymphocyte. These *in vitro* studies need to be interpreted within the broad perspective of the development and function of the immune system *in vivo*. A number of studies imply that the hormonal milieu *in vivo* plays an important role in modulating the performance of the cellular immune system and in maintaining its integrity. The pituitary, adrenal and thyroid glands[9] and both the parasympathetic and sympathetic limbs of the autonomic nervous system[10] would appear to be important participants in such a modulatory role. Each of these endocrine and neural systems has been related in one way or another to intracellular cyclic nucleotide messenger systems. The *in vitro* experiments then should be interpreted as demonstrating, in a highly selective way, the roles the two cyclic nucleotides may play in lymphocyte metabolism and proliferation. Their interpretation with respect to the intact *in vivo* system must be restricted in two senses: first, the *in vivo* milieu provides a myriad of influences, potentially operant in a concomitant manner through the cyclic nucleotide systems such that a synthetic response might be expected to result; and, second, the lymphocyte, as it moves through its developmental process, would logically be envisioned to demonstrate an evolving and changing sensitivity to various hormonal agents.

Before exploring these molecular aspects of cellular immunity, I would like to briefly summarize certain developmental and functional aspects of the cellular immune system. The "T" cell finds its origin in a stem cell derived within the bone marrow and sharing ancestry with other cells of the hematopoietic system. This cell traffics via the peripheral blood to the thymus where it continues to proliferate until it undergoes a complex differentiation process. This process is presumably mediated by the specific microchemical environment of this central lymphoid organ, very likely through the action of one or more thymic hormones. The differentiation process involves a cessation of proliferation and the acquisition of certain distinctive cell surface markers and ultimately of the ability to bind and to respond to antigen and to certain plant lectins such as phytohemagglutinin (PHA) and Concanavalin A (Con A). The differentiated thymocyte then traffics to the peripheral blood and lymphatic system when it continues to recirculate. On response to antigenic stimulation, this lymphocyte responds with three distinct but interrelated functions. It proliferates to expand the sensitized population. It liberates a number of soluble mediators which modulate the function of macrophages (macrophage migration inhibitory factor, aggregating factor, activating factor and chemotactic factor) and of granulocytes (polymorphonuclear and eosinophil chemotactic factors) and which participate in anti-viral defense (interferon) and anticellular responses (lymphotoxin). In addition, it may participate in a direct cytotoxic interaction with foreign cells, either malignant or engrafted (lymphocytotoxicity response). These three major responses, once triggered, run their course and result in long lived memory cells capable of reinstituting the process upon re-exposure to the same antigen.

The characteristic of the "T" lymphocyte to bind and to respond to plant mitogens, such as PHA and Con A, has provided an important tool for the study of these cells in culture. When stimulated by these mitogens, large populations of these "T" lymphocytes proliferate, produce soluble mediators and kill target cells in a manner indistinguishable from the process induced by specific antigen.

The earliest studies of cyclic nucleotides and lymphocytes employed these mitogens and involved study of the proliferative response of lymphocytes in culture. A number of workers, including ourselves,[11-14] added to phytohemagglutinin stimulated lymphocyte cultures a variety of agents designed to increase cellular cyclic AMP levels and found the subsequent DNA synthesis suppressed. Others[13] observed that control cultures without phytohemagglutinin were unaffected or slightly stimulated by such additions to the culture. These early experiments served to support the concept emerging at that time from data in a number of systems that increases in cellular cyclic AMP were somehow antiproliferative in their effect.

Further manipulations ensued in which agents were administered to increase cyclic AMP levels in proliferating lymphocytes specifically during the induction period ("Go" or early "G_1") and during the period of most active DNA synthesis ("S" phase).[14,15] It was found that increases in cyclic AMP induced by β adrenergic agents antagonized PHA induction of proliferation but enhance DNA synthesis once in progress. Concomitant studies of changes in glucose uptake, glycogen content and lactate production[15,16] indicated that at least in part, the increased cyclic AMP levels were associated with alterations in glucose utilization comparable to those observed in other tissues (i.e., increased glycogen breakdown and depressed glucose uptake). These studies

175

imply that cyclic AMP functions in the lymphocyte as in the liver to activate glycogenolysis through the now well established protein kinase-glycogen phosphorylase activation sequence. The cyclic AMP mediated alterations in PHA-induced DNA synthesis may have resulted from manipulations of glycogen metabolism antagonistic to those naturally occurring following induction; however, as will be mentioned later, other possible intracellular actions of cyclic AMP might also account for the observed effects. The pertinent conclusion derived from these observations is that metabolic events initiated by phytohemagglutinin, such as glycogen accumulation and DNA synthesis, are consistent with the absence of cyclic AMP action and that events promoted by cyclic AMP are antagonistic to mitogen induction of proliferation.

Further studies of lymphocyte proliferation have provided insights into what role cyclic GMP plays in this process. Following on the observation of George *et al.*[3] suggesting cyclic GMP might be involved in a cholinergic mediator mechanism, we studied the effects of acetylcholine on lymphocyte cyclic GMP levels[2] and on PHA induced transformation.[7,17] We found that acetylcholine, acting through a muscarinic receptor mechanism increases cyclic GMP levels (three-fold) in the lymphocyte without significant effect on cyclic AMP levels and has an associated effect to augment PHA-induced RNA, protein and DNA synthesis. These studies serve to contrast β adrenergic and cholinergic modulation of lymphocyte proliferation and to associate cyclic AMP with inhibition and cyclic GMP with stimulation of the proliferative response.

Within this framework, a number of hormonal agents can now be considered as having action to modify lymphocyte proliferation through one or the other of the two cyclic nucleotide systems. Prostaglandin E_1[18] and perhaps glucagon and histamine (unpublished observations) have been observed to inhibit lymphocyte proliferation and have been shown[19] or are expected, based on their action in other systems, to have their effect through cyclic AMP. Certainly other hormones and hormonal agents will be added to this list in the near future.

Alpha adrenergic stimulation, like cholinergic stimulation, is associated with augmentation of PHA-induced lymphocyte transformation.[14] This action, not clarified *vis a vis* cyclic nucleotides in the nucleotides in the lymphocyte, has been associated with increases in cyclic GMP[4,7] and a lowering of cyclic AMP in several tissues.[19] In addition, alpha adrenergic effects to stimulate membrane transport adenosine triphosphatases (ATPases) have been reported,[20] effects which may, on the basis of recent evidence, be related to effects of cyclic nucleotides on transport.

Another hormone, not yet clarified in its mechanism of action, is insulin.

The evidence for the presence of insulin receptors on lymphocytes is controversial[21,22] and would appear to depend upon the method of isolation. Similarly, the effects of insulin on lymphocyte ATPase, cyclic GMP levels, transport and metabolism are controversial for apparently the same reason.[22–25] One interpretation of these findings is that methods yielding virtually pure "T" cells indicate a lack of each of these responses[22,25] associated with no effect of insulin on PHA-induced "T" cell proliferation (unpublished data). In contrast, studies employing methods yielding both "T" and "B" lymphocytes or pure "B" lymphocytes indicate the presence of insulin receptors[21] and insulin effects to increase membrane ATPase,[23] cyclic GMP levels,[24] transport and metabolism.[23,24] These findings taken in conjunction with our initial observation[7,8] that insulin increases cyclic GMP in fibroblasts and the recent observation of Illiano et al.[25] that insulin increases cyclic GMP levels of fat and liver cells indicate that cyclic GMP is central to insulin action and that the action of insulin on lymphocytes is restricted to the antibody-producing "B" lymphocytes.

The findings that a variety of hormones, and hormone-like agents, modulate lymphocyte proliferation through apparent mediation of the cyclic nucleotides have provided a basis for extending these observations to other lymphocyte functions as well as to other cells involved in the immune response. The process by which lymphocyte mediators are produced by sensitizing "T" cells on exposure to antigen is augmented by cholinergic stimulation to increase cyclic GMP levels[7] and suppressed by agents which increase cyclic AMP levels.[26] Similarly, the process of target cell killing (lymphocytotoxicity) is augmented by increasing cellular cyclic GMP[27] and inhibited by increasing levels of cyclic AMP.[27,28] Others[7] have provided evidence for similar modulation of macrophage migration, leukocyte degranulation, mast cell and basophil histamine release and platelet aggregation, evidence which underscores the ubiquity of these modulation processes in cells of the hematopoietic, lymphoid and reticuloendothelial systems.

The discussion to this point has centered upon how hormonal agents act and how they modify lymphocyte metabolism and proliferation induced by mitogens or antigens; of perhaps greater importance is how mitogens and antigens themselves activate lymphocytes to perform their functions of proliferation, mediator production and cytotoxicity. Considerable evidence supports the concept that antigens and mitogens interact with surface receptors and some evidence[30] indicates that the mitogens need not enter the cell to induce cellular division. This evidence supports the hypothesis[6] that mitogens trigger cell division by a discrete activation of the cell membrane and employ cyclic nucleotide mechanisms much the way hormones do.

This concept derives from studies of the mechanisms by which PHA and Con A induce proliferation in lymphocytes. Despite previous conflicting studies concerning an action of PHA to increase cellular cyclic AMP levels in lymphocytes[18,30-32] our own studies[6] have indicated that while unpurified PHA may have a slight action to increase lymphocyte cyclic AMP levels, purified PHA or Con A have no effect to alter the levels of cyclic AMP.

Additionally, we observed that both PHA and Con A produce striking (10-50 fold) increases in lymphocyte levels of cyclic GMP. These increases were rapid and discrete (30 min.) and occurred whether or not purified mitogens were used. The profile of the cyclic AMP response corresponded to that of PHA binding and suggested the involvement of cyclic GMP is a trigger type of signal mechanism. Although these increases occur in association with a number of other changes in membrane function[6] we are predisposed for several reasons to consider the cyclic AMP increase and the associated early influx of calcium to be central to the process of induction of cell division.

The concomitant increase in calcium influx is considered to be of central importance because of the general importance ascribed to calcium in cellular proliferation,[33] its demonstrated early influx in PHA-stimulated but not in acetylcholine-stimulated lymphocytes,[34,17] its required presence during the induction phase[35] and certain observations to be discussed concerning its relationship to the intracellular action of cyclic GMP.

The cyclic GMP increase is considered by us to be central for two reasons. The first rests upon evidence derived from studies in other systems in which the induction of proliferation by hormones and mitogens has been studied. In one system in particular, the hypothesis had been previously advanced[36,37] that cyclic AMP levels are essential to the regulation of proliferation in that high levels inhibit and lowered levels are associated with induction of proliferation. Our own studies[7,8,38] indicate that several agents (insulin, serum and phorbol myristate acetate) which induce proliferation in confluent mouse fibroblasts produce striking early increases in cellular cyclic AMP levels. These observations support our original contention[6] that a temporally discrete rise in cellular cyclic GMP levels represent an active signal to induce proliferation while changes in cyclic AMP levels are associated with regulatory influences which limit or inhibit proliferation. This hypothesis has found direct support in recent evidence from a variety of systems in which proliferation has been induced;[38a-d] it has received indirect support in those observations which indicate that in rapidly proliferating cells cyclic GMP levels are increased and cyclic AMP levels generally unchanged or lowered.[8,24,39,40] This latter support is considered indirect as it has been shown that cyclic AMP levels change during the cell cycle[41] and we have preliminary evidence that cyclic GMP levels also vary with the cell cycle. The interpretation of averaged levels in non-synchronized cell populations is, therefore, limited. These cell cycle-related changes imply changing roles for the cyclic nucleotides during the cell cycle and may serve to explain why, during the latter phases of the cell cycle, influences which increase cyclic nucleotide levels have differing effects on DNA synthesis and on the progression of cells to mitosis.

The second line of reasoning supporting a role for cyclic GMP as an intracellular messenger involved in the induction of lymphocyte proliferation rests upon observations of the effects of cyclic GMP on RNA synthesis in isolated lymphocyte nuclei.[8,17] Among the earliest changes following mitogen interaction with lymphocytes are those which occur within the nucleus. These include the stimulation of histone acetylation,[42] nuclear protein phosphorylation,[43] RNA polymerase activity[44] and nuclear RNA synthesis.[42] Our studies on the effects of low concentrations of cyclic GMP (10^{-10} M range) to stimulate RNA synthesis in isolated nuclei in the presence of calcium indicate that cyclic GMP and calcium are reproducing the effect of PHA on the nucleus of the intact cell and, therefore, appear to be the mediators of a cell surface-to-nuclear mitogenic signal. Considerable work will be required to clarify these events; however, they serve to suggest that an intranuclear action of cyclic GMP may be an important aspect of its intracellular action.

Little more can be said about possible sites of biochemical action of cyclic GMP within the lymphocyte. Recent studies imply that the well known effects of insulin to induce glucogen accumulation in liver through an activation of the glycogen synthetase pathway can be related to observed increases in cyclic GMP[25] and suggest that PHA and alpha adrenergic effects to increase glycogen content of the lymphocyte[15,16] will be similarly mediated by cyclic GMP effects on this pathway.

Despite more than ten years of intensive study of cyclic AMP, relatively little can be said about the possible intracellular actions of this cyclic nucleotide in the lymphocyte. As indicated, we have observed the activation of glycogenolysis by agents which increase lymphocyte cyclic AMP levels, an action presumably mediated by the mechanisms to activate phosphorylase worked out in liver. We[8,17] have also observed effects of cyclic AMP at high concentrations (10^{-6} M) to induce RNA synthesis in isolated lymphocyte nuclei, an effect which may relate to similar observations in liver,[45] perhaps mediated by the effects of cyclic AMP to activate a histone kinase and induce histone phosphorylation.[46]

With intracellular action of the cyclic nucleotides restricted presently to regulation of glycogen and of not yet understood nuclear events, considerable work in the future will be required to clarify the role of the cyclic nucleotides as mediators of a large variety of environmental influences (e.g., steroid hormones) acting through mechanisms not perhaps directly involving the cyclic nucleotides.

Still a third perspective in which the cyclic nucleotides are to be appreciated as playing a role concerns the development of the "T" lymphocyte from the marrow-derived stem cell precursor. Although not demonstrated, one might envision the existence of a "poietin" growth factor, much like erythropoietin, which would act at the marrow level, perhaps only early in life, to induce proliferation of the "T" cell precursor in order to provide the requisite seeding and subsequent replenishment of the cellular components of this system. Within the perspectives herein outlined, we would presume such a growth factor would act to increase cyclic GMP in such precursor cells. As mentioned, as this cell traffics to the thymus, it rapidly proliferates. Within this circumstance, the participation of cyclic nucleotides and calcium in the regulation of proliferation of thymus cells have been shown by the extensive investigation of Whitfield, MacManus and their coworkers.[33] The relationship of cyclic AMP, cyclic GMP and calcium in influencing proliferating thymocytes is complex and, in some aspects, apparently paradoxical. A simple interpretation of these observations is that a rapidly dividing subset of thymocytes is subject to a large variety of hormonal influences and that agents which increase cyclic AMP enhance the flow of cells into mitosis when the exposure occurs during the latter phases of the cell cycle. An agent presumed to increase cyclic GMP[47] and cyclic GMP itself[48] inhibit this process. Not accounted for by this simple interpretation, is the reversal of cyclic nucleotide effects by the manipulation of extracellular calcium concentration.[33] While a definitive explanation is not possible at this time, these works are convincing in demonstrating that these cells have a broad spectrum of hormonal sensitivity and that both cyclic nucleotides play a role in modulating the proliferation of cells already engaged in the process.

As these dividing presursor cells are induced to become mature thymocytes they cease proliferating and gain a number of surface and functional characteristics. Recent evidence[49–51] suggests that the thymus gland elaborates one or more hormonal factors which in semipurified form will induce in precursor cells from marrow or spleen the acquisition of several of the surface and functional traits characteristic of the mature "T" cell. The action of the hormone(s) has been indirectly related to cyclic AMP in that cyclic AMP itself and agents which increase cyclic AMP will mimic the effect of the hormone. While definitive proof is lacking (experiments in progress), the existence of a differentiative antiproliferative thymus-derived hormone which acts through cyclic AMP is, indeed, attractive to explain in part the mechanisms of development within this system. Clearly, the door has only just opened on what must be many influences acting within this system whose elucidation will provide a basis for understanding and manipulation of cellular immune response.

It is of note that two adjuvants, poly A-poly U and endotoxin,[51] which have been observed to increase cyclic AMP in these or similar cells,[30,52] mimic the thymus hormone action, thus suggesting a mechanism by which these agents enhance immune response. The extensive work of Braun and his associates [53,54] on the action of Poly A-U to increase T-dependent B-cell responses *in vivo* and *in vitro* may ultimately find their explanation in its action to increase cyclic AMP in thymus precursors, thus enhancing their differentiation into contributors, either directly or through released factors,[51] to the "T" helper function necessary for "B" antibody production.

Based on these pioneering, yet unfulfilled steps toward an understanding of hormone, mitogen and adjuvant action within the cellular immune system, the future would appear bright in terms of eventual clarification of the mechanisms of action, both cellular and subcellular, of a large number of agents acting within this system. The understanding of the roles played by cyclic nucleotides in biologic regulation provides a basis for anticipation and predicting not only the mechanism of action of biologically active hormonal factors based on the cellular responses observed but also for predicting where pharmacologic manipulation may be effective in influencing cellular proliferation and immune function.

Speculation

The observation that agenesis of the immune system with abrogation of immune response, both cellular and hormonal (Cf. proceedings of this Symposium), relates to a deficiency of adenosine deaminase (ADA) raises the speculation that somehow the cyclic nucleotides are involved. Although this enzyme deficiency is closely related to the pathways involved in cyclic nucleotide metabolism (See Fig. 1), no experimental data exists to implicate the cyclic nucleotides directly or indirectly in mediating the antilymphocyte effects of this deficiency.

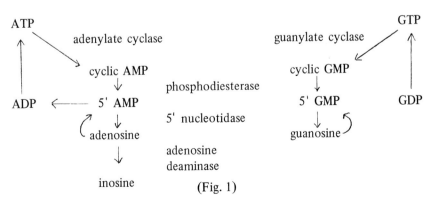

(Fig. 1)

To date, the demonstration of an ADA defect in all cells of affected individuals in the presence of essentially normal development and function of all systems except for the immunologic, implies an extraordinary sensitivity on the part of the lymphocyte to the results of the deficiency. Although the basis for the sensitivity is not known, the works of R. Hirschhorn and H. Green, presented at this conference, suggest that accumulation of adenosine could be involved. If so, this accumulation could provide an influence by which cyclic nucleotide levels, particularly cyclic AMP levels, might be increased and lymphocyte proliferation blocked.

An alternative hypothesis is that the genetic defect in ADA deficiency involves several genes on the same chromosome and the ADA gene defect is therefore linked to a defective locus responsible for immune development and/or response.

Summary

Cyclic AMP and cyclic GMP appear to be mediators of hormonal and of proliferative influences acting in thymus-related and thymus-dependent lymphocytes. Hormonally-induced increases of lymphocyte cyclic AMP levels are associated with *inhibition* of the induction of proliferation, of the secretion of soluble mediators and of lymphocytotoxicity and with *enhancement* of the process of proliferation of actively dividing lymphocytes and GMP levels are associated with the *augmentation* of the induction of proliferation in lymphocytes and lymphocyte precursors. Hormonally-induced increases of lymphocyte cyclic GMP levels are associated with the *augmentation* of the induction of proliferation in lymphocytes, of soluble mediator production and lymphocytotoxicity and with *inhibition* of actively dividing lymphocyte precursors. Hormone-like substances acting to induce differentiation in thymocyte precursors are tentatively concluded to act through cyclic AMP. Mitogenic agents acting to induce proliferation in differentiated thymocytes are tentatively concluded to act through cyclic GMP. The cellular metabolic responses induced by cyclic AMP imply an intracellular action to induce glycogenolysis and an intranuclear action to regulate RNA synthesis. The cellular metabolic responses induced by cyclic GMP imply an intracellular action to induce glycogen synthesis and an intranuclear action to regulate RNA synthesis (presumably by different mechanisms than those regulated by cyclic AMP). The collected evidence suggest complex and complementary roles of the cyclic nucleotides in mediating a large variety of regulatory influences, hormonal and other, on lymphocyte differentiation, proliferation and function. Any direct relationship between ADA deficiency, cyclic nucleotides and lymphogenesis remains to be determined.

REFERENCES

1. N.D. Goldberg, R. O'Dea and M.K. Haddox,Recent Advances in Cyclic Nucleotide Research, Vol. 3, Raven Press, New York, 1973.

2. N. Goldberg, M. Haddox, D. Hartle and J. Hadden, *Proc. V. Int. Congress Pharmacol. 5,* 146, 1973.

3. W.J. George, J.B. Polson, A.G. O'Toole and N.D. Goldberg, *Proc. Nat. Acad. Sci. 66,* 398, 1970.

4. G. Schultz, J.G. Hardman, J. Davis, K. Schultz and E.W. Sutherland, *Fed. Proc. 31,* 440, 1972; *Proc. Nat. Acad. Sci. 70,*1721, 1973.

5. J. Kuo, T. Lee, P.L. Reyes, K.G. Walton, T.E. Donnelly and P. Greengard, *J. Biol. Chem. 247,* 16, 1972.

6. J. Hadden, E. Hadden, M. Haddox and N. Goldberg, *Proc. Nat. Acad. Sci. 69,* 3024, 1972.

7. N.D. Goldberg, M.K. Haddox, C. Lopez, R. Estensen and J.W. Hadden, Cyclic AMP Immune Response and Tumor Growth, Springer-Verlag, New York, 1973. (In press)

8. N.D. Goldberg, M.K. Haddox, E. Dunham, C. Lopez and J.W. Hadden, Cold Spring Harbor Symposium, Control of Proliferation in Animal Cells, 1973. (In press)

9. J. Comsa, *in* Thymic Hormones, University Park Press, Baltimore, 1973.

10. J. Hadden and W. Summerlin, *Proc. II Int. Congress of Psychomatic Medicine,* Amsterdam, 1973. (In press)

11. C. May, *J. Allergy 43,* 163, 1969.

12. J.W. Smith, A. Steiner, W.M. Newberry and C.W. Parker, *Fed. Proc. 28,* 566, 1969.

13. R. Hirschhorn, J. Grossman and G. Weissman, *Proc. Soc. Exp. Biol. Med. 133,* 1361, 1970.

14. J.W. Hadden, E.M. Hadden and E. Middleton, *J. Cell Immunol. 1,* 583, 1969.

15. J.W. Hadden, E.M. Hadden and R.A. Good, *Biochem, Biophys. Acta 237,* 1971.

16. J.W. Hadden, E.M. Hadden, E. Middleton and R.A. Good, *Int. Arch. Allerg. and Immunol. 40,* 526, 1971.

17. J.W. Hadden, E.M. Hadden, G. Meetz, R.A. Good, M.D. Haddox and N.D. Goldberg, *Fed. Proc. 32,* 1022, 1973.

18. J.W. Smith, A.L. Steiner and C.W. Parker, *J. Clin. Invest. 50,* 442, 1971.

19. E.W. Sutherland, G.A. Robinson and R.W. Butcher, *Circulation 37,* 279, 1968.

20. J. Hadden, E. Hadden and R. Coffey, *Fed. Proc. 30,* 687, 1971; R.G. Coffey, J.W. Hadden, E.M. Hadden and E. Middleton, *Fed. Proc. 30,* 497, 1971.

21. J.R. Gavin, J. Roth, P. Jen and P. Freychet, *Proc. Nat. Acad. Sci. 69,* 747, 1972.

22. V. Krug, F. Krug and P. Cuatrecasas, *Proc. Nat. Acad. Sci. 69,* 2604, 1972.

23. J.W. Hadden, E.M. Hadden, E.E. Wilson, R.A. Good and R.G. Coffey, *Nature, New Biol. 235,* 174, 1972.

24. J.W. Hadden and N.D. Goldberg (unpublished observations).

25. G. Illiang, G.P.E. Tell, M.I. Siegel and P. Cuatrecasas, *Proc. Nat. Acad. Sci. 70,* 2443, 1973.

26. B. Bloom (preliminary unpublished observations).

27. T. Strom, A. Deisseroth, J. Morgan, C.B. Carpenter and J.P. Merrill, *Proc. Nat. Acad. Sci. 69,* 2995, 1972.

28. C.S. Henney and L.M. Lichtenstein, *J. Immunol. 107,* 610, 1971.

29. M.Greaves and S. Bauminger, *Nature, New Biol. 235,* 67. 1972.

30. R. Winchurch, M. Ishizuka, D. Webb and W. Braun, *J. Immunol. 106,* 1399, 1971.

31. A. Novogradsky and E. Katchalski, *Biochem. Biophys. Acta 215,* 291, 1971.

32. M.K. Makman, *Proc. Nat. Acad. Sci. 68,* 885, 1971.

33. J.F. Whitfield, R.H. Rixon, J.P. MacManus and S.D. Balk, *In Vitro 8,*

257, 1963.

34. G. Allwood, G.L. Asherson, M.J. Davey and P.J. Goodford, *Immunol.* *21,* 509, 1971.

35. R.B. Whitney and R.M. Sutherland, *J. Cell Physiol. 80,* 329, 1973.

36. J.R. Sheppard, *Nature, New Biol. 236,* 14, 1972.

37. J. Otten, G.S. Johnson and I. Pastan, *J. Biol. Chem. 247,* 7082, 1972.

38a. R.D. Estensen, J.W. Hadden, E.M. Hadden, M.K. Haddox and N.D. Goldberg, Cold Spring Harbor Symposium, Control of Proliferation in Animal Cells, 1973. (In press)

   b. A. Valeri, E.J. Ruoslalti and T. Hovi, *ibid.*

   c. H. A. Armelin, K. Nishikawa and G.H. Sato, *ibid.*

   d. J. Voorhees, M. Stawiski, E. Duell, M. Haddox and N. Goldberg, *ibid.*

39. J. Voorhees, M. Stawiski, E. Duell, M. Haddox and N. Goldberg, *Life Science II,* 1973. (In press)

40. E.W. Thomas, F. Murad, W.B. Looney and H.P. Morris, *Biochem. Biophys. Acta 297,* 564, 1973.

41. M. Burger, B. Bombik, B. Breckenridge and J.R. Sheppard, *Nature, New Biol. 239,* 161, 1972.

42. B.G.T. Pogo, V.G. Allfrey and A.E. Mirsky, *Proc. Nat. Acad. Sci. 55,* 805, 1966.

43. L.J. Kleinsmith, V.G. Allfrey and A.E. Mirsky, *Science 154,* 780, 1966.

44. B.G.T. Pogo, *J. Cell Biol. 53,* 635, 1972.

45. J.P. Jost and M.K. Sahib, *J. Biol. Chem. 246,* 1623, 1971.

46. T.A. Langan, *in* Role of Cyclic AMP in Cell Function, Raven Press, New York, 1970.

47. J.P. MacManus and J.F. Whitfield, *Endocrinology 86,* 934, 1970.

48. J.F. Whitfield and J.P. MacManus, *Proc. Soc. Exp. Biol. and Med. 139,* 818, 1972.

49. J.F. Bach, M. Dardenne and M. Bach, *Transplant. Proc. 5,* 99, 1973.

50. K. Komuro and E.A. Boyse, *Lancet I,* 740, 1973.

51. M.P. Shied, M.F. Hoffman *et al., Lancet,* 1973. (In press)

52. M. Bitensky, R. Gormon and L. Thomas, *Proc. Soc. Exp. Biol. and Med. 138,* 773, 1971.

53. M. Ishizuka, W. Braun and T. Matsumoto, *J. Immunol. 107,* 1027, 1971.

54. M. Ishizuka, M. Gafni and W. Braun, *Proc. Soc. Exp. Biol. and Med. 134,* 963, 1970.

DISCUSSION

MARTIN B. VANDERWEYDEN (Duke University Medical Center, Durham, North Carolina): Has Dr. Green measured the phosphoribosyl pyrophosphate (PRPP) levels in the cell lines he exposed to pharmacologic concentrations of adenosine and has he measured the orotic acid phosphoribosyl transferase (OPRTase) and PRPP synthetase activities in these cells?

DR. GREEN: PRPP levels are down somewhat.

DR. VANDERWEYDEN: Do you get the same effect by exposing the cells to the same concentration of hypoxanthine?

DR. GREEN: No, hypoxanthine and adenine do not produce this form of toxicity up to 1.0 mM.

DR. VANDERWEYDEN: Didn't Dr. Krooth publish (*Cold Spring Harbor Sym. Quant. Biol. 29,* 189, 1964) that the effect of adenosine in fibroblasts derived from patients who were heterozygous or homozygous for congenital orotic aciduria was to inhibit growth of these cell lines so that the induced effect of adenosine would occur in the absence of or substantially reduced levels of OPRTase and orotidylic decarboxylase (ODCase) activities?

DR. GREEN: Krooth showed that adenosine slowed the growth of homozygous mutant cells. It didn't kill them.

DR. VANDERWEYDEN: Didn't this effect occur in the presence of uridine or cytidine?

DR. GREEN: Uridine or cytidine relieved the inhibition. I discussed this with Dr. Krooth and it seems likely that the reason wild type cells were not affected is that most of the added adenosine was destroyed by adenosine deaminase in the serum supplement. The mutant cells are probably more sensitive to traces of adenosine.

DR. VANDERWEYDEN: Has anybody ever seen megaloblastic hemopoiesis in patients with CID?

DR. POLLARA: As far as I know, only Dr. Pickering's patient may be having problems. I didn't mean to imply that patients with hereditary orotic aciduria were immunodeficient. I don't think they have been worked up from this point of view but the first recorded case did die from a varicella infection.

DR. PICKERING: This patient is complicated. She has received plasma and required transfusions. I think that is due to the fact that we are repeatedly drawing blood from her. For the past two or three weeks, her red blood cells (smears) were somewhat bizarre looking with a variation of cell size and a lot of target cells. We have just done a bone marrow and I haven't yet learned the results. Dr. Rosen has had a lot of experience with these patients. I don't know if he has ever seen a megaloblastic anemia in them. This patient, in addition, has a lot of problems with malabsorption. She has been on folic acid, vitamins and iron but we have not treated her with vitamin B_{12} until recently.

DR. POLLARA: Dr. Glasky, I don't know whether I was surprised or not to see normal adenosine levels in the red cells of Dr. Pickering's case but where do you think the adenine comes from?

DR. GLASKY: There is no phosphorylase in the erythrocytes and I think it is something we should look at. Whether this has actually been determined or not, I think the only place it can come from is adenosine.

DR. PARKS: Several colleagues of mine at Brown University (T.P. Zimmerman, N.B. Gersten, A.F. Ross and R.P. Miech, *Can. J. Biochem.* 49, 1051, 1971) have examined the reactivity of adenine with purine nucleoside phosphorylases from various sources, including a preparation of the crystallized human erythrocyte enzyme prepared in my laboratory. They have reported that the K_m value for adenine is about 4×10^{-4} M which is about 20 times greater than the K_m value for hypoxanthine. However, the V_{max} for ribosylation of hypoxanthine was about 1600 times greater than that for adenine. Therefore, it appears that erythrocytic purine nucleoside phosphorylase has only weak reactivity with adenine and adenosine. However, one should bear in mind that the activity of purine nucleoside phosphorylase in human erythrocytes (about 10 μmolar units per ml of cells) is about one hundred fold greater than the activity of adenosine deaminase, so that the phosphorolysis of adenosine might become significant under conditions where adenosine deaminase is deficient or inhibited. Recently, Snyder and Henderson (*J. Biol. Chem.* 248, 5899, 1973) have shown that in the presence of the potent adenosine deaminase inhibitor coformycin, human erythrocytes can cleave deoxyadenosine to form adenine.

I would like to comment on Dr. Green's paper. There is evidence from our laboratory (Nelson and Parks, *Cancer Research 23,* 1034, 1972) and from Paterson's laboratory at the University of Alberta (Warnick and Paterson, *Cancer Research 33,* 1711, 1973) which indicates that an analog of adenosine, 6-methylmercaptopurine ribonucleoside (MMPR), can stimulate rather than inhibit the synthesis of pyrimidine ribonucleotides in Sarcoma 180 ascites cells and Lymphoma L5178Y cells. MMPR is not a substrate for purine nucleoside phosphorylase, is a relatively weak inhibitor of ADA but is an excellent substrate for adensoine kinase in a variety of tissues and readily forms the 5′-monophosphate ribonucleotide. Therefore, this monophosphate nucleotide is a very poor substrate for adenylate kinase and di- and triphosphate nucleotide (MMPR-P) can accumulate in cells, including tumor cells, and the half time for degradation of MMPR-P in tumor cells is 14 hours or more. This analog mononucleotide, as shown by Hill and Bennett, is a very powerful feedback inhibitor of PRPP-amido transferase, the first step in the de novo synthesis of purines. This potent and long-sustained inhibition of de novo purine biosynthesis results in a marked increase (5 to 10 fold) in the steady-state levels of PRPP in cells. For reasons as yet unexplained, although the synthesis of MMPR-P with inhibition of de novo purine biosynthesis occurs rapidly (30 to 60 minutes), the increase in the steady-state level of PRPP is delayed and reaches a peak in 6 to 12 hours. The inhibition of de novo purine biosynthesis results in a marked fall in the purine nucleotide levels of cells. On the other hand, reactions catalyzed by the purine salvage enzyme, HGPRTase, are enhanced probably as a result of the greater availability of PRPP. Also, presumably as a result of the higher PRPP levels, the intracellular concentrations of the pyrimidine nucleotides, UTP and CTP, approximately double. These observations suggest that the availability of PRPP plays an important role in determining the rate of pyrimidine nucleotide synthesis (since PRPP is required for the formation of orotidylate from orotate). It looks as though there may be competition between the various metabolic pathways for the PRPP. This suggests the possibility that the toxicity of adenosine discussed by Dr. Green could be due to effects on PRPP availability and perhaps the enzyme, PRPP synthetase. Studies from a number of laboratories indicate that PRPP synthetase is an important site for regulatory mechanisms.

DR. GREEN: That is interesting and does sound like a regulation type of effect. In our experiments, if we add up the total orotate and uridine nucleotides that are made in the presence of adenosine, it is not decreased; it's more than in the control. Adenosine doesn't shut off the entire pyrimidine pathway, it just prevents the last stages of the pathway.

189

DR. PARKS: The key factor may be the steady-state level of PRPP. If that falls dramatically under your conditions, it would explain the failure of orotate to form orotidylate.

DR. VANDERWEYDEN: The importance of measuring OPRTase and ODCase activities is that if adenosine does cause a serial depletion of PRPP then this might shut off carbamyl phosphate synthetase (CAP Synth.) activity because it has been established by Japanese workers (Tatibana *et al., Advances in Enzyme Reg. 10,* 249, 1972) that the first enzyme in the pyrimidine de novo pathway, CAP Synth., is activated by PRPP and inhibited by UTP. There is also some evidence that the first three and last two enzymes in the pyrimidine de novo pathway exist in complexes. (Shoaf and Jones, *Biochemistry 21,* 4039, 1973). Regulation of the stability of these complexes in the pyrimidine de novo pathway might well revolve around the intracellular PRPP levels.

DR. KEIGHTLEY: In support of Dr. Green's suggestion that uridine might be used to treat these patients, I'd like to present some preliminary findings with platelets from the parents of the affected child and of the child himself. We've been particularly interested in looking at platelets because here you have a situation where platelets contain storage granules of adenosine diphosphate and during the process of platelet aggregation ADP is released into the surrounding plasma. ADP has been shown to be broken down to adenosine and then degraded to inosine then hypoxanthine.

Any adverse effect that might result from decreased degradation of adenosine might affect platelet function and one easy way of studying this is to look at platelet rich plasma in an aggregometer. This simply measures changes in optical density as a function of time. Normally, platelet aggregation in response to agents such as adrenalin occurs in a biphasic manner. You get a primary wave of aggregation induced by the agent, followed by a secondary wave of aggregation as platelet ADP is released. In the three family members I have mentioned, we've only been able to find the primary wave of aggregation. This has been on repeated occasions when we took particular care to make sure they were not taking aspirin or any other pharmacological agent that might inhibit aggregation in normal people. After we heard of Dr. Green's findings we were able to obtain a normal secondary wave following incubation with 1 mM uridine for one hour at room temperature.

HANS OCHS (University of Washington, Seattle, Washington): During this meeting an effort was made to explain why ADA deficiency causes combined immune deficiencies. Dr. Rochelle Hirschhorn presented data demonstrating a qualitative change of adenosine deaminase in lymphocytes during PHA, Con-A and pokeweed mitogen stimulation. Our laboratory studied the quantitative changes of adenosine deaminase activity during lymphocyte stimulation with PHA, Con-A, pokeweed mitogen and PPD. The lymphocytes were obtained from a PPD positive individual.

Lymphocyte cultures stimulated with PHA showed a marked increase of ADA activity between 5 and 10 days following addition of PHA. The enzyme activity per one million cells could not be determined because of massive clumping of the lymphocytes.

Figure 1 demonstrates the situation in the Con-A stimulated culture. The abscissa shows the time of incubation in days; the ordinate shows the different parameters studied (e.g., cell number, H^3-thymidine, ADA activity in mμmoles/hr/10^6 cells). The cell number of the non-stimulated cultures remains stable until day 6 then declines rapidly. The ADA activity of the non-stimulated cultures remains stable until day 6 then declines rapidly. The ADA activity of the non-stimulated controls also remains stable and persists for 10 days. Two days after Con-A is added, thymidine is incorporated rapidly and peaks by day 5 with a stimulatory index of 80. Thereafter H^3-thymidine incorporation declines rapidly. The adenosine deaminase activity per million cells rises continuously beginning at day 5, reaching a maximum at day 10 (4 to 5 times the activity of the control).

Figure 2 portrays the situation in the PWM stimulated culture. Thymidine incorporation occurs later and cell number increases less rapidly and later than in the Con-A stimulated cultures. ADA activity per million cells did not increase until day 9 and 10 when marked increase was apparent.

Figure 3 shows the changes during PPD stimulation. The increase of cell number and the incorporation of H^3-thymidine occurs later than in cultures stimulated with nonspecific antigens and no increase of ADA activity was observed.

These studies would indicate that ADA activity per lymphocyte increases significantly during stimulation with Con-A and to a lesser extent during stimulation with pokeweed mitogen. The increase of lymphocyte ADA activity occurs after the maximum H^3-thymidine incorporation is over. One would expect that if ADA is important for DNA synthesis, the increase of lymphocyte ADA activity would precede the H^3-thymidine incorporation.

KURT HIRSCHHORN: Did you change medium during this 10 day period at all?

DR. OCHS: No. We used 10% fetal calf serum in our medium and washed

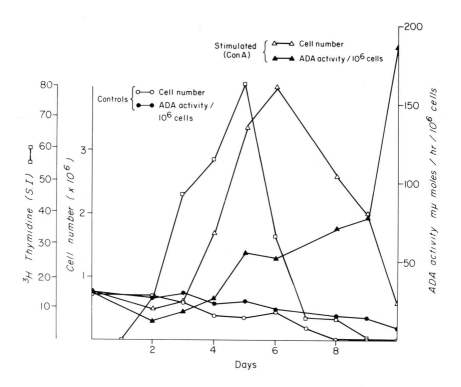

Fig. 1.

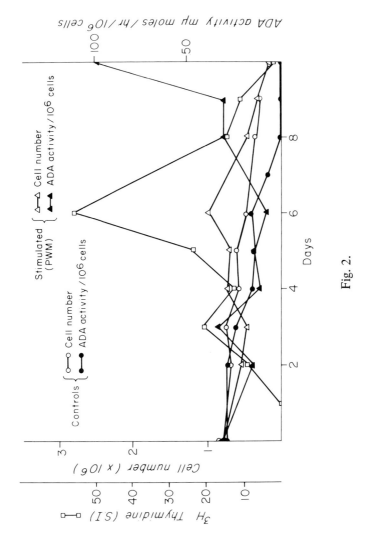

Fig. 2.

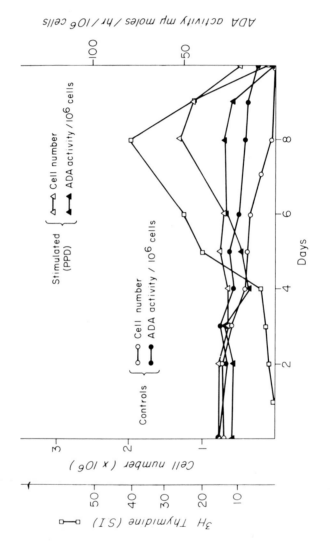

Fig. 3.

194

the cells carefully after harvesting them.

KURT HIRSCHHORN: The only suggestion I have to explain your results, and I think this could be tested fairly easily, is that in the proliferating cultures, mainly with Con-A, in which you got this very late, enormous rise in ADA activity, there may be something in the medium that was depleted. In turn, ADA activity was induced in these cells rather than increased as a response to the stimulation. The timing seems so far removed that one suspects some secondary effect.

DR. OCHS: A lot of cells died, especially in the cultures stimulated with Con-A. We also noticed that the pH became markedly acid and I think your suggestion will be pursued further.

DR. PARKS: For the past few years our laboratory has been studying human erythrocytic adenosine deaminase and we have developed a relatively simple isolation procedure that permits several thousand fold purification of the enzyme in reasonably good yields from large quantities of blood. We have recently completed a study of the kinetic parameters of the natural substrates, adenosine and deoxyadenosine, as well as of a number of nucleoside analogs, and a manuscript describing this work is under review (R.P. Agarwal, S.M. Sagar and R.E. Parks, Jr., *Molec. Pharmacol.* Submitted for publication).

Table 1 presents the K_m and relative V_{max} values for some of these compounds. Note that the K_m of adenosine is about 25 μmolar whereas with 2'-deoxyadenosine the K_m is about three fold lower. Also of interest is the K_m of arabinosyladenine which is about five fold higher than that of adenosine. This suggests an important role for the 2'-position of the ribose moiety in substrate binding. Two of the analogs of considerable interest are formycin A (a C-nucleoside) and 8-azaadenosine. Both of these analogs are modified in the imidazole position of the purine ring and have diazo linkages in the 7 and 8 positions. Although these compounds have higher Michaelis constants than adenosine, they react with the enzyme much more rapidly as is shown by the elevated V_{max} values. Also of interest are the analogs tubercidin (7-deazaadenosine), 2-fluoroadenosine and 2-fluorodeoxyadenosine which are devoid of substrate activity. In a study reported recently from this laboratory (Parks and Brown, *Biochemistry 12,* 3294, 1973) on the incorporation of various adenosine analogs into the nucleotide pools of human erythrocytes, it was seen that incubation of these cells with adenosine and deoxyadenosine did not significantly modify the adenine nucleotide pools but rather caused an accumulation of inosinic acid. Also, incubation with formycin A did not lead to the formation of formycin nucleotides. However, several analog nucleo-

TABLE 1

Kinetic Constants of Human Erythrocytic Adenosine Deaminase

Substrate	Km $(M \times 10^5)$	Relative Vmax
Adenosine	2.5	100
2'-Deoxyadenosine	0.7	60
Xylofuranosyl Adenine	3.3	62
Arabinofuranosyl Adenine	10.0	47
4'-Thioadenosine	1.3	43
3'-Deoxyadenosine	4.1	110
3'-Amino-3'-deoxyadenosine	13.3	89
Formacin A	100.0	800
8-Azaadenosine	13.0	310
6-Chloropurine ribonucleoside	100.0	91
2,6-Diaminopurine ribonucleoside	7.4	91

sides that are incapable of reacting with adenosine deaminase, such as tuberci-din, N^6-methyl adenosine and 2-fluoroadenosine, entered the nucleotide pools readily and formed large amounts of analog nucleotides. In fact, the concentrations of 2-fluoroATP formed after two hours of incubation exceeded the normal concentration of ATP in the erythrocyte by several fold. Presumably this indicates that these compounds are capable of reacting with adenosine kinase in the erythrocyte.

Table 2 presents the results of studies of inhibition of ADA by several adenosine analogs. All of the inhibitors listed gave classical patterns of competitive inhibition on Lineweaver-Burke plots. Of interest is the relatively potent inhibition seen with 2-fluoroadenosine and 2-fluorodeoxy adenosine which indicates that these compounds can bind to the active site without undergoing deamination. On the other hand, tubercidin is devoid of inhibitory activity. Of special interest and of great potential for future studies of the role of adenosine deaminase in cellular metabolism is the inhibitor coformy-cin, discovered by Dr. Hamao Umezawa and his colleagues. Although the structure of this inhibitor has not yet been reported, it is an N-nucleoside with a molecular weight and chemical composition similar to adenosine (Empiric formula $C_{11}H_{16}N_4O_5$). This compound is an inhibitor of adenosine deaminases from a variety of sources and we have found that it is a tight-binding inhibitor of erythrocytic ADA with a K_1 value of about 0.01 μmolar. This important new ADA inhibitor is available in only small quantities and we are grateful to Professor Umezawa for giving my colleague, Dr. Senft, a few milligrams. When larger amounts become available, coformycin could become an important tool for evaluating the significance and role of adenosine deaminase in tissue metabolism. It is possible that many of the biochemical features seen in cells from patients with the combined immunological deficiency syndrome considered at this Symposium could be mimicked by incubation of cells with coformycin. For example, one might predict that adenosine might enter the adenine nucleotide pools more readily rather than being converted to inosinic acid. Also, inhibitors such as formycin A that are rapidly deaminated by ADA might more readily form analog nucleotides in the presence of coformycin. We have recently offered an hypothesis (Parks and Brown, *Biochemistry 12,* 3294, 1973) concerning the control mechanism for the decision of whether adenosine is salvaged in cells by the reaction with adenosine kinase or degraded to inosine by adenosine deaminase. It was proposed that the balance between the activities of these two enzymes and their relative Michaelis constants is the crucial factor. Cells from patients deficient in adenosine deaminase could provide a unique opportunity to test this hypothesis. Of course, we also hope to challenge this hypothesis in experiments with coformycin.

TABLE 2

Inhibition Constants of Human Erythrocytic Adenosine Deaminase

Inhibitors	K_1 $(M \times 10^5)$
Inosine	11.6
Deoxyinosine	6.0
Guanosine	14.0
2-Fluoroadenosine	6.0
2-Fluorodeoxyadenosine	1.9
N'-Methyladenosine	27.5
N^6-Methyladenosine	1.7
6-Thioinosine	33.0
6-Methylthioinosine	27.0
6-Thiopurine-arabinoside	41.0
6-Thioguanosine	9.2
Coformycin	0.001
N^7-Methylinosine	>> 100
N^7-Methylguanosine	>> 100
Tubercidin	>> 100
Toyocamycin	>> 100

An important facet of purine nucleotide metabolism not considered at this Symposium is the transport of these compounds into the cell. Paterson's group (Cass and Paterson, *J. Biol. Chem.* *247,* 3314, 1972) has demonstrated the presence of a facilitated transport system for nucleosides such as adenosine. This system is highly active but may be inhibited by certain nucleoside analogs. One wonders whether defects in this transport mechanism might also result in deficits in the functioning of lymphocytes.

EFFECTOR PHASE ABNORMALITIES OF CELL MEDIATED IMMUNITY IN FAMILY MEMBERS OF A CHILD WITH HEREDITARY T CELL IMMUNODEFICIENCY AND ABSENT ADENOSINE DEAMINASE*

Flossie Cohen
James J. Lightbody**

Human peripheral blood lymphocytes sensitized by allogeneic cells in the one-way mixed leukocyte culture (MLC) are rendered specifically cytotoxic to lymphocytes autologous to the sensitizing cells.[1] This cell-mediated lympholysis (CML) is thought to represent the efferent phase and the MLC the afferent phase of the allograft rejection. A recent adaptation described by Lightbody *et al.*[2] has greatly increased the applicability of CML and is based on the observation that PHA stimulated lymphocytes become sensitive targets for effector lymphocytes previously sensitized in MLC. A first requisite for effective destruction in CML is the activation of responding cells by stimulator cells in the MLC prior to their becoming the effector cells in the CML. A second requisite for effective destruction in CML is a difference in the serologically defined antigens of the major histocompatibility complex, HL-A in man and H-2 in the mouse, between the stimulator and responder in MLC and a similar difference between the effector and target in CML. The second requisite was described from studies done in the mouse[3] and from family studies done in humans,[4] and suggests that once lymphocytes are activated in MLC, the serologically defined antigens determine the extent of CML.

This report concerns the results of MLC and CML assays done on family members of a child with a major hereditary immunodeficiency and with absent adenosine deaminase.[5] The father and mother and some of the relatives showed reduced to absent CML despite MLC activation and despite disparity in the serologically defined antigens of the HL-A complex. This suggests a selective defect in the efferent phase of the allograft rejection in the parents and other family members of this patient.

*Supported by N.I.H. Grant No. HD00505 and American Cancer Society I.C. 82.

**Assistant Professor of Biochemistry, Wayne State University, Detroit, Michigan.

Materials and Methods

Lymphocytes were obtained from heparinized peripheral blood separated on a Ficoll-Hypaque gradient (sp. gr. 1.077) as described by Boyum.[6] The MLC was done by the method of Solliday and Bach.[1] Into 16 x 100 mm glass tubes were put $1.5x10^6$ responding and $1.5x10^6$ stimulating cells in a total volume of 2 ml of tissue culture medium 199 supplemented with penicillin (100 U/ml), streptomycin (100 μg/ml) and 20% frozen human pooled plasma. (TC 199-20). Stimulator cells were treated with mitomycin-C (25 μg/ml), incubated for 20 minutes at 37°C in 95% air and 5% CO_2. Five days later, 0.2 ml aliquots were put in Linbro microculture plates with 2 μ Ci of tritiated thymidine (Schwarz-Mann, sp. act. 1.19 units) and incubated for 12 hours. The cells were then precipitated on glass fiber filters using the procedure of Hartzman et al.[7] and counted in a Packard scintillation counter. All reactions were done in duplicate. The remainder of the responding cells from the MLC provided the effector cells for the CML. The target cells were prepared in parallel with the MLC. These were incubated in TC-199-20 ($1x10^6$ lympho-cytes/ml) in Falcon plastic bottles (Falcon 3040) for three days, at which time PHA (1:100 dilution PHA-M, Difco Laboratories) was added. After three additional days in culture; i.e., on day 6, they were centrifuged (200 x g) for 10 minutes and suspended in 0.3 ml of TC-199-20 (approximately 8 x 10^6 cells) and were labeled with 150 μ Ci of Na $^{51}CrO_4$ (New England Nuclear). The mixture was incubated for one hour with frequent shaking at 37°C, washed twice with TC-199-20 in the cold and resuspended at 1 x 10^5 cells/ml.

For the cytotoxicity assay, 0.1 ml containing 1 x 10^6 effector cells (based on viable cells, determined by eosin dye exclusion) and 0.1 ml containing 1 x 10^4 target cells were placed in round bottom Linbro microculture plates, which were incubated for 4 hours at 37°C in 95% air and 5% CO_2. The micro-plates were centrifuged (100 x g) for 10 minutes and an aliquot removed and counted. The actual test release of ^{51}Cr reflecting the degree of killing of the target cells by the effector cells is derived from the formula $\frac{E - S}{T - S}$ x 100, E representing the experimental release of ^{51}Cr, S the spontaneous release (target cells incubated alone) and T the total release from the same number of target cells after freezing and thawing. Thus, E - S reflects the degree of killing of the effector cells and T - S is the maximum amount of chromium available to demonstrate cell destruction.

When significant killing occurs, controls establishing the specificity of the killing are needed. Responder cells are added to mitomycin-C treated autologous cells in the MLC, and are then reacted with allogeneic target cells. Killing may occur and generally yields up to 10% ^{51}Cr release. We, therefore, consider 0-10% ^{51}Cr release as negligible or non-significant and greater than 10% ^{51}Cr release as significant. While 10-20% ^{51}Cr release is considered significant, it is also considered low cytotoxicity, since the majority of normal individuals affect a release generally greater than 20% ^{51}Cr. A further control, necessary when significant killing has occurred, is the exclusion of the spurious form of "autokilling". For this, effector cells previously stimulated by allogeneic cells in the MLC are challenged in CML with cells autologous to the effector cells. When no significant killing is demonstrated in CML, it is necessary to exclude the possibility that inherent characteristics of the target cell precludes killing. This is accomplished if killing occurs when the effector cells other than the test subjects are used.

Results

Both the history and study of genetic markers failed to demonstrate any evidence of consanguinity in this family. The pedigree, ABO and HL-A* types are shown in Fig. 1. None of the members including the parents are HL-A identical and they differ from each other for at least two serologically determined antigens.

Table 1 shows the results of the MLC and CML when the mother's (M) lymphocytes were tested as responder and stimulator in the MLC and as effector and target in the CML. The mother as responder (effector) showed negligible to low cytotoxicity towards the father's lymphocytes on four different occasions despite stimulation in the MLC. In addition, cytotoxicity, though slightly better towards the lymphocytes of the four unrelated individuals (A_1, A_2, A_3, A_4), was still defective and the mean of all her responses was 11.6 $\pm$ 7.1% compared to the mean of 26 normals, which was 41.3 $\pm$ 21.7% with a p-value of 0.001. Additionally, lymphocytes from the father's parents were also used as target cells for the mother as responder (effector) and the cytotoxicity was negligible.

The father, like the mother, responded poorly in the CML when both the mother's lymphocytes and those of unrelated individuals were the targets (Table 2). The mean of all his responses was 13.14 $\pm$ 7.9%, with p 0.01. Here again, there was negligible cytotoxicity when lymphocytes from the mother's parents were used as targets.

While it is accepted that the MLC response is prerequisite for efficient CML, no exact correlation has been established between the degree of response in MLC and the degree of response in CML. Of the four unrelated individuals used, the lymphocytes belonging to A_3 were most easily killed by both parents, despite a lack of increase in the level of stimulation in the corresponding MLC. This shows that the precise relationship of factors affecting the susceptibility to killing in CML and the ability to stimulate in MLC are as

*We are grateful to Dr. Kissmeyer-Nielson for the HL-A typing of those family members other than the propositus.

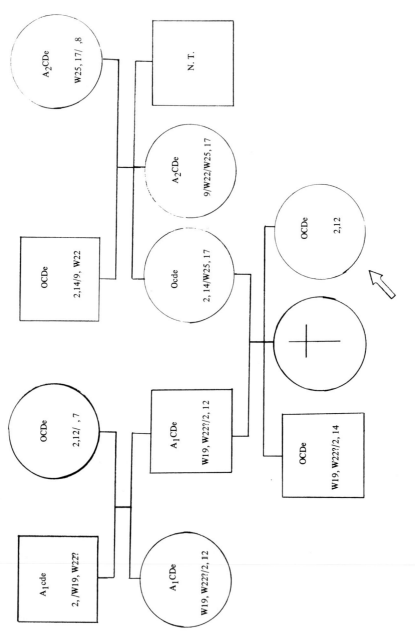

Fig. 1. Pedigree with ABO, Rh, and HL-A types

204

TABLE 1

MLC and CML – PATIENT'S MOTHER

RESPONDER (effector) STIMULATOR	MLC ^{3}HT UPTAKE MEAN cpm ± S.D.				TARGET	CML ^{51}Cr RELEASE MEAN cpm ± S.D.								p value*
	Exp. 1 cpm ± S.D.	Exp. 2 cpm ± S.D.	Exp. 3 cpm ± S.D.	Exp. 4 cpm ± S.D.		Exp. 1 cpm Percent ± S.D.		Exp. 2 cpm Percent ± S.D.		Exp. 3 cpm Percent ± S.D.		Exp. 4 cpm Percent ± S.D.		
M/F	21,777 ± 537	7,427 ±1,715	23,916 ± 348	22,080 ± 141	F	1,409 ± 25	2.4	2,917 ± 113	1.5	2,605 ± 91	6.3	1,163 ± 16	19.3	
M/M	971 ± 106	858 ± 89	1,552 ± 114	1,643 ± 64	F	1,337 ± 30	- 4.5			1,043 ± 46	- 4.3			
M/A1	13,462 ± 245				A1	1,343 ± 177	10.6							
M/A2		14,628 ± 157		21,003 ±1,188	A2			2,264 ± 64	6.7					
M/A3			18,263 ± 541	11,972 ±4,943	A3					1,978 ± 30		763 ± 96	22.8	
M/A4				19,646 ±17,872	A4							944 ± 83	15.6	p = 0.001

The percent ^{51}Cr release is based on the following spontaneous release (SR) and maximum release (MR) for each target cell in each experiment (mean ± S.D. of duplicates).
F (father): exp. 1 SR=1,384± 21, MR=2419± 14; exp. 2 SR=2891± 71, MR=4821± 28; exp. 3 SR=2368± 29, MR=6089± 321; exp. 4 SR=908± 55, MR=2256± 64.
A1 (unrelated adult): exp. 2 SR=2181± 88, MR=3552± 134; exp. 4 SR=1083± 24, MR=1994± 156.
A2 (unrelated adult): exp. 3 SR=1357± 14, MR=3584± 54; exp. 4 SR=419± 25, MR=1994± 40.
A4 (unrelated adult): exp. 4 SR=665± 45, MR=2453± 210.

*26 normal adults: 41.3 ± 21.7.

TABLE 2

MLC and CML – PATIENT'S FATHER

RESPONDER (effector) STIMULATOR	MLC 3HT UPTAKE MEAN cpm ± S.D.				TARGET	CML 51Cr RELEASE MEAN cpm ± S.D.				p value
	Exp. 1 cpm ± S.D.	Exp. 2 cpm ± S.D	Exp. 3 cpm ± S.D.	Exp. 4 cpm ± S.D.		Exp. 1 cpm Percent ± S.D.	Exp. 2 cpm Percent ± S.D	Exp. 3 cpm Percent ± S.D.	Exp. 4 cpm Percent ± S.D.	
F/M	4,535 ± 146	7,958 ± 1,260	7,852 ± 159	15,220 ± 2,335	M	2,055 13.1 ± 161	1,682 7.2 ± 23	1,038 - 4.8 ± 8	1,071 20.1 ± 87	
F/F	1,338 ± 153	931 ± 15	822 ± 97	2,101 ± 37	M	1,563 - 4.7 ± 112	1,502 - 4.1 ± 16	1,054 - 3.2 ± 60	900 0.8 ± 55	
F/ A1	8,799 ±1,935				A1	1,177 1.8 ± 94				
F/ A2		10,932 ± 671		20,073 ± 580	A2		2,392 15.1 ± 40		1,580 18.3 ± 39	
F/A3			8,662 ± 656	22,172 ±3,760	A3			1,749 16.7 ± 60	793 30.1 ± 82	
F/A4				23,969 ±4,164	A4				883 12.2 ± 47	p = 0.01

The percent 51Cr release is based on the spontaneous release (SR) and maximum release (MR) for each target cell (mean ± S.D. of duplicates). M (mother): exp. 1 SR=1659± 27, MR=4430± 7; exp. 2 SR=1570± 51, MR=3125± 84; exp. 3 SR=1084± 44, MR=2018± 430; exp. 4 SR=728± 10, MR=2134± 46.

Refer to Table 1 for SR and MR of target cells A1, A2, A3, A4.

206

yet unknown.

As a result of these findings in the parents, we studied CML in other members of this family and Table 3 shows the responses of the father's mother (FM), the father's father (FF) and the father's sister (FS), when tested against the lymphocytes of unrelated individuals A_2, A_3 and A_4. Again, cytotoxicity was poor, though less poor than for the parents, with p-values of < 0.05. The findings in the mother's family (Table 4), from tests on the mother's mother (MM), the mother's father (MF), the mother's sister (MS) and her son (S); i.e., the patient's brother, showed that even though all, except the mother's mother, had p-values greater than 0.05 and are statistically insignificant, they belong in the lower end of the normal spectrum.

In contrast, Table 5 shows the composite results of unrelated individuals A_1, A_2 and A_3 tested with the lymphocytes of different family members as targets. Repeated testing of the same individual with different targets consistently gave normal results and clearly demonstrated that lymphocytes of the family members were susceptible to killing. In addition, cells of another unrelated adult, A_5, were used as the effector, and the lymphocytes of A_2, A_3 and A_4 as targets, to demonstrate their cellular susceptibility to killing. The findings clearly demonstrate that A_2, A_3 and A_4 were capable of being killed when the effector lymphocytes belonged outside the family.

Discussion

The mixed lymphocyte culture, considered to represent the afferent phase of the allograft rejection, has been shown to be independent of the sero-logically defined antigens.[8] Thus, adequate stimulation in the MLC is possible in the absence of HL-A differences between responder and stimulator, establishing an independent genetic control for MLC and HL-A. On the other hand, CML, considered to represent the efferent phase of the allograft rejection, has been shown to be dependent upon MLC stimulation and, in addition, to be dependent upon HL-A differences between effector and target.[3,4] Thus, effector cells stimulated in MLC direct their killing toward the serologically defined antigens on the target cells.

In this family of a patient with a major hereditary immunodeficiency and ADA deficiency, the members had both the necessary requisites – MLC activation and HL-A disparity for CML. However, despite these requisites, there was abnormal to absent CML on repeated testing, which suggests a defect in the effector phase of allograft rejection.

While the precise relationship between CML and MLC is still relatively unclear, evidence suggests that CML and MLC are mediated by separate cell populations.[9] The dichotomy observed between MLC activation and CML in this family would be compatible with either the concept that separate cell

TABLE 3

MLC and CML – FATHER'S PARENTS and SISTER

RESPONDER (effector) STIMULATOR	MLC ^{3}HT UPTAKE MEAN cpm ± S.D. Exp. 2 cpm ± S.D.	Exp. 3 cpm ± S.D.	Exp. 4 cpm ± S.D.	TARGET	CML ^{51}Cr RELEASE MEAN cpm ± S.D. Exp. 2 cpm Percent ± S.D.	Exp. 3 cpm Percent ± S.D.	Exp. 4 cpm Percent ± S.D.	p value
FM/A2	7,439 ±1,447		10,766 ± 954	A2	2,478 21.3 ± 52		1,137 2.0 ± 16	
FM/FM	1,356 ± 16		1,909 ± 272	A2	2,148 - 2.5 ± 19			
FM/A3		12,255 ± 628	17,411 ± 356	A3		16,505 13.1 ± 60	991 36.3 ± 52	p = <0.05
FM/FM		469 ± 162	1,909 ± 200	A3		1,322 - 1.6 ± 20	656 - 0.6 ± 14	
FM/A4			11,452 ±1,252	A4			910 13.7 ± 33	
FM/A2	7,869 ±2,520		26,050 ±2,034	A2	2,177 - 0.3 ± 32		1,113 1.1 ± 118	
FF/FF	1,284 ± 21		1,745 ± 441	A2	2,006 -12.4 ± 124		1,021 - 2.3 ± 68	
FF/A3		15,694 ± 895		A3		1,723 16.4 ± 35		
FF/FF		1,152 ± 71		A3		1,342 - 0.8 ± 20		
FF/A4			27,556 ±1,566	A4			823 8.8 ± 108	p = <0.05
FS/A2			14,699 ±2,266	A2			1,304 8.2 ± 35	
FS/A3			12,453 ±3,453	A3			667 15.7 ± 52	
FS/FS			1,244 ± 130	A3			421 0.1 ± 11	
FS/A4			18,112 ± 66	A4			903 13.3 ± 75	p = <0.05

The percent ^{51}Cr release is based on the spontaneous release (SR) and maximum release (MR) for each target cell (mean ± of duplicates). FM = father's mother, FF = father's father, FS = father's sister.

Refer to Table 1 for SR and MR of target cells A1, A2, A3, A4.

TABLE 4

MLC and CML – PATIENT'S BROTHER, MOTHER'S PARENTS and SISTER

RESPONDER (effector) STIMULATOR	MLC ^{3}HT UPTAKE MEAN cpm ± S.D.		TARGET	CML ^{51}Cr RELEASE MEAN cpm ± S.D.		p value
	Exp. 4 cpm ± S.D.			Exp. 4 cpm ± S.D.	Percent	
MM/A$_2$	12,453 ±4,353		A$_2$	1,593 ± 14	18.9	
MM/A$_3$	5,802 ± 332		A$_3$	1,173 ± 655	16.1	
MM/MM	608 ± 3		A$_3$	381 ± 45	- 2.4	
MM/A$_4$	17,904 ±1,998		A$_4$	839 ± 124	9.7	p = 0.05
MF/A$_2$	7,320 ± 578		A$_2$	1,300 ± 279	17.3	
MF/A$_3$	17,928 ± 916		A$_3$	1,284 ± 301	34.7	
MF/A$_4$	14,966 ±2,646		A$_4$	821 ± 74	14.3	
MF/MF	1,071 ± 191		A$_3$	422 ± 17	0.2	p = 0.09
MS/A$_2$	14,279 ±1,683		A$_2$	1,213 ± 16	4.8	
MS/A$_3$	7,729 ± 147		A$_3$	884 ± 45	29.5	
MS/MS	1,108 ± 256		A$_3$	457 ± 71	2.4	
MS/A$_4$	18,556 ±1,120		A$_4$	1,273 ± 12	34.0	p = 0.07
S/A$_2$	19,553 ± 156		A$_2$	1,149 ± 113	2.3	
S/S	2,303 ± 430		A$_3$	421 ± 8.4	0.1	
S/A$_4$	19,122 ±5,121		A$_4$	1,014 ± 77	19.5	p = 0.06

MF = mother's father, MM = mother's mother, MS = mother's sister, S = son (brother of propositus).

The percent ^{51}Cr release is based on the spontaneous release (SR) and maximum release (MR) for each target cell (mean ± S.D. of duplicates).

Refer to Table 1 for S.R. and M.R. of target cells A$_1$, A$_2$, A$_3$, A$_4$.

209

TABLE 5

MLC and CML – UNRELATED CONTROLS

RESPONDER (effector) STIMULATOR	MLC ^{3}HT UPTAKE MEAN cpm ± S.D. cpm ± S.D.	TARGET	CML ^{51}Cr RELEASE MEAN cpm ± S.D. cpm ± S.D.	Percent
A_1/F	36,384 ±1,529	F	1,858 ± 80	43.8
A_1/F		A_1	1,208	- 8.1
A_1/M	10,569 ± 681	M	2,428 ± 6	26.5
A_1/A_1	3,363 ± 465	M	1,186 ± 4	2.3
A_1/M		A_1	1,182 ± 58	2.1
A_2/M	13,543 ± 193	M	2,255 ± 57	44.0
A_2/A_2	361 ± 83	M	1,495 ± 23	4.5
A_2/F	9,468 ± 358	F	3,631 ± 33	47.2
A_2/A_2		F	2,765 ± 2	- 6.1
A_2/FM	19,972 ±1,365	FM	3,187 ± 50	67.4
A_2/FF	20,192 ± 67	FF	3,291 ± 60	46.2
A_3/M	24,206 ± 501	M	1,494 ± 31	44.1
A_3/A_3	1,654 ± 157	M	1,013 ± 6	- 7.4
A_3/F	26,087 ± 368	F	3,998 ± 5	44.0
A_3/A_3		F	2,272 ± 41	- 2.5
A_5/A_2	15,946 ± 161	A_2	2,222 ± 56	42.4
A_5/A_3	23,062 ±1,393	A_3	1,040 ± 83	39.4
A_5/A_4	19,586 ±1,348	A_4	1,232 ± 282	31.7
A_5/A_5	995 ± 105	A_2	1,126 ± 40	1.6
A_2/A_3	38,510 ±5,159	A_2	490 ± 38	3.2
A_3/A_2	25,906 ± 137	A_3	487 ± 120	4.3
A_4/A_2	17,704 ±4,784	A_4	741 ± 105	4.1

The percent ^{51}Cr release is based on the spontaneous release (SR) and maximum release (MR) for each target cell (mean ± S.D. of duplicates).

FM = father's mother, SR = 2405, MR = 3560; FF = father's father, SR = 2533, MR = 4170.

Refer to Table 1 for SR and MR of other target cells.

populations mediate MLC and CML, or the concept that a single cell population mediates MLC and CML, because the data could represent a selective functional defect within one cell population. The role of ADA in the immune system and the effects of its interaction with other gene products is not known. The proposita had severe immunodeficiency combined with absent ADA, had B cells determined by their ability to form "EAC" rosettes and essentially normal B cell function; had normal numbers of T-lymphocytes determined by their ability to form "E" rosettes and had a defect of T cell function, which suggests a relationship between ADA activity and T cell function. This relationship gains support from the findings of the parents, who are apparently healthy adults, heterozygous for ADA (with decreased but not absent levels of ADA) and in whom only selective and not total T cell defect is demonstrated by the abnormal CML.

Even if this relationship between ADA and CML were to be established in the parents, it would not explain the generally low responses observed in other members of the family. Since the importance of the age factor in CML is unknown, abnormality in the grandparents might be influenced by it. Although for the other family members the statistically insignificant, but nonetheless low-normal responses remain unexplained, the observations would suggest the interaction of a variety of unusual genes on both sides of this family resulting in *in vitro* functional aberrations in the family members and in lethal immunodeficiency in the proposita and her sister. Even the apparently homozygous state in the two siblings was considerably different in its phenotypic expression, which supports the concept of multiple gene interactions.

Thus, in this rather unique family with two children afflicted with major immunodeficiency and ADA deficiency, the repeatedly abnormal CML found in the parents, serves as a distinguishing feature of the heterozygous state.

REFERENCES

1. S. Solliday and F.H. Bach, *Science 170*, 1406, 1970.

2. J.J. Lightbody, D. Bernaco, V.C. Miggiano and R. Ceppellini, *G. Batteriol. Virol. Immunol. 64*, 273, 1971.

3. B.A. Alter, D.J. Schendel, M.L. Bach, F.H. Bach, J. Klein and J.H. Stimpfling, *J. Exp. Med. 137*, 1303, 1973.

4. V.P. Eijvoogel, R. duBois, C.V.M. Melief, W.P. Zeylemaker, L. Ratt-Koning and L. de Groot-Kooy, *Transplant. Proc. 5*, 415, 1973.

5.   E.R. Giblett, J.E. Anderson, F. Cohen, B. Pollara and H.J. Meuwissen, *Lancet 2,* 1067, 1972.

6.   A. Boyum, *Scand. J. Clin. Lab. Invest. (Thesis) 21,* 1968.

7.   R.J. Hartzman, M. Segall, M.L. Bach and F.H. Bach, *Transplant. Proc. 2,* 268, 1971.

8.   E.J. Yunis and D.B. Amos, *Proc. Natl. Acad. Sci. 68,* 3031, 1971.

10. F.H. Bach, M. Segall, K.S. Zier, P. Sondel, B. Alter and M. Bach, *Science 180,* 403, 1973.

CORRECTION OF COMBINED IMMUNODEFICIENCY BY FETAL LIVER TRANSPLANTATION IN A PATIENT WITH ADENOSINE DEAMINASE DEFICIENCY*

R.G. Keightley
A.R. Lawton
L.Y.F. Wu
M.D. Cooper

Definitive treatment of severe combined immunodeficiency by bone marrow transplantation has been limited to the minority of patients possessing histocompatible donors. When these have not been available, transplantation of unmatched marrow has regularly been followed by fatal graft versus host disease. Reduction in the number of grafted cells, differential separation procedures, graft pretreatment with anti-lymphocyte serum or maintenance chemotherapy of the recipient have either not been successful in preventing graft versus host disease or have prevented engraftment. In one instance, treatment with maternal plasma possessing a unique blocking factor led to prolonged recipient survival following a maternal bone marrow graft but for the majority of these patients, no effective treatment has been previously available (reviewed by Buckley).[1]

An alternative to the physical separation of presumptive lymphoid stem cells from immunocompetent lymphocytes has been to take advantage of the ontogeny of lymphoid development and utilize hemopoietic cells obtained from fetal liver before the attainment of immunocompetence. Prolonged recipient survival and lack of graft versus host disease has been noted following reconstitution of irradiated rodents with allogeneic fetal liver.[2]

Having made the diagnosis of SCID in a boy with no potential marrow donor, we decided to treat him with fetal liver. His sister had died at two months of age with meningitis, pneumonia, oral candidiasis and otitis media. At autopsy she had shown severe lymphoid hypoplasia, with no Peyer's patches or gut-associated lymphoid tissue, few lymphocytes in the spleen and only a rudimentary thymus. A few Hassall corpuscles were present.

*Supported by Grants RR 3213, Al CA 11502-01, CA 13148-02 from the U.S.Public Health Service and the American Cancer Society, Alabama Division.

213

Forwarned by this family history, we were able to study our patient from birth using previously described methods for the enumeration of T cells by the E rosette technique,[3] and of B cells by staining for surface immunoglobulins.[4] The cord blood showed an extreme deficiency of cells bearing surface immunoglobulins with only a very rare cell (3 in about 100,000 scanned) positive for IgM. Subsequently, on repeated occasions he lacked any cells having the morphological appearance of lymphocytes or any cells bearing IgM, IgA or forming rosettes with sheep cells. Cord serum contained a trace of IgM that persisted for the first 6 weeks of life but then became undetectable.

Screening examination of a red cell lysate kindly performed by Dr. B. Pollara at one month of age showed an absence of red cell adenosine deaminase. Reduced enzyme activity has been found in his father and several paternal relatives. The mother, however, falls within the lower limits of the normal range. X-rays of the patient showed flared costochondral junctions, widened metaphyses and a dysplastic pelvis.

At the time of transplantation, at three months of age, he had no detectable serum IgM or IgA, and had no B-lymphocytes bearing μ or a determinants, no rosette forming cells and no *in vitro* response to mitogens.

He was then given 2×10^8 viable cells from the liver of a 9 week fetus by intra-peritoneal injection. Nineteen days later the first IgM positive cell was seen. One week later, serum IgM was detected and a few E rosettes were noted.

By 39 days, the lymphocyte count was 300 per cubic millimeter, 19% formed E rosettes, 8% had surface IgM and an occasional cell was positive for IgA.

The absolute number of T cells then increased rapidly as shown in Fig. 1 but normal numbers have not yet been achieved. A positive response to PHA was first found on the 74th day. Subsequently, significant proliferative responses have been obtained to Concanavalin A, Candida antigen and mitomycin treated allogeneic lymphocytes in mixed lymphocyte culture.

Serum IgM stayed low until 84 days post transplant when it rose rapidly to 200 mg% then fell to normal levels. Six months post transplantation a titer of 1:128 was obtained following 3 immunizations with typhoid vaccine Seven months post transplant at 10 months of age, he weighs 16 pounds. His absolute lymphocyte count is 1000. 7% have surface IgM and 1% have surface IgA. Serum IgM is 46 mg%, IgG 370 mg%, IgA 15 mg%.

Lymphocyte HLA typing has been performed on both sets of parents. The patient's own father has 2, 7 and 3, 7 haplotypes; his mother has 2, 5 and 9, W22 haplotypes. Both the father and mother of the fetus have HLA 2 and W28 in the first series and W5 in the second series. Five and a half months post transplantation, the donor antigen W5 was found on peripheral blood

CORRECTION OF COMBINED IMMUNODEFICIENCY IN AN ADENOSINE DEAMINASE
DEFICIENT INFANT BY FETAL LIVER (9 weeks) TRANSPLANTATION

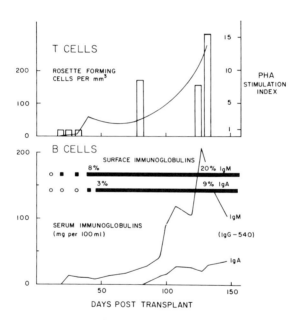

Fig. 1

215

lymphocytes establishing the existence of a chimeric state.

Eighty-four days post transplant normal adenosine deaminase activity was found in lymphocytes and could also be detected in serum. Enzyme activity has risen much more slowly in red cells reaching only 4% of normal by 150 days. However, this value is in keeping with evidence for red cell chimerism. Three to 5% of his red cells possess the Kidd antigen Jk[a] which was not found prior to transplant and is lacking in his parents but possessed by the father of the fetus.

This is the first successful repair of severe combined immune deficiency by fetal liver transplantation. At 9 weeks of gestation, this organ contains only a very rare cell bearing surface IgM determinants.[5] Proliferative responses to allogeneic lymphocytes have been found as early as ten weeks of gestation[6] but these cells are unresponsive to mitogens. The significance of this finding is not clear in regard to their potential to produce clinical graft versus host disease. Our patient had a transient rash fifty days post transplantation but skin biopsy did not support a diagnosis of graft versus host disease. Given the above evidence for chimerism, our presumption is that we have given stem cells, free of significant contamination by immunocompetent lymphocytes, which have developed into functioning T and B cells tolerant of the host. If this interpretation is correct, the adequacy of thymic and bursal micro-environments to serve as induction sites in this kind of immune deficiency is established. A further possibility in this particular patient is that transfer of normal cells producing adenosine deaminase has facilitated the development of his own as well as donor lymphocytes. Analysis of this situation by differential *in vitro* cell killing is in progress.

The absence of severe graft versus host disease and the continuing good health of this patient suggests that transplantation with fresh liver from fetuses less than 12 weeks of age deserves serious consideration in the treatment of children with SCID lacking compatible donors.

REFERENCES

1. R.H. Buckley, *in* Progress in Immunology 1 (B. Amos, Ed.), p. 1061, Academic Press, New York, 1971.

2. D.E. Uphoff, *J. Nat. Cancer Inst. 20,* 625, 1958.

3. M. Jondal, G. Holm and H. Wigzell, *J. Exp. Med. 136,* 207, 1972.

4. M.D. Cooper, A.R. Lawton and D.E. Bockman, *Lancet II,* 791, 1971.

5. A.R. Lawton, K.S. Self, S.A. Royal and M.D. Cooper, *Clin. Immunol. Immunopath. 1,* 104, 1972.

6. M.C. Carr, D.P. Stites and H.H. Fudenberg, *Nature New Biol.* *241,* 279, 1973.

SCREENING FOR ADA DEFICIENCY *

Ellen C. Moore
Hilaire J. Meuwissen

Recently it has been shown that some forms of combined immuno-deficiency disease (CID) are associated with deficient activity of the enzyme adenosine deaminase (ADA).[1-4] ADA deficiency (ADAD) is potentially detectable at birth, whereas CID is usually not diagnosed until the onset of infections. Earlier detection of CID by ADA assay would greatly benefit these patients, particularly if a histocompatible marrow donor were available. ADAD appears to be fairly specific for CID: only one possible case in a normal person[5] has been detected so far in several thousand people screened, whereas the 12 other known cases of ADAD have all had CID.[6] Assessment of the true incidence of this deficiency though will require the testing of a far greater number of persons.

The usual methods for measuring ADA are too laborious for large scale screening however and, furthermore, require venous blood which is not readily available from newborns. We have therefore developed a screening method adopted from Ressler's[7] technique in which we use a drop of blood spotted on filter paper identical to the samples routinely used in screening newborns for metabolic disorders. Three sixteenths of an inch discs are punched from the dried blood spots and placed on a gel containing the reagents. This gel is prepared by mixing bromthymol blue (Sigma, saturated solution in normal saline), 5 ml, and adenosine (Baker grade, J.T. Baker, 0.02 M in normal saline), 91.3 ml, and combining this with 100 ml of melted agarose, 2% in normal saline pH 6.0. It is important that glassware and other materials in contact with the reagents be rinsed thoroughly prior to use to remove any alkali residue. The mixture is kept liquid at 45° C while the wells of a dispotray (Model 96 SC clear plastic, Limbro, 96 cups, 5 ¾" x 8") are filled level with the top using a prewarmed repeating syringe. Then, after the gel has hardened, the filter paper blood spots are pressed firmly on the gel surface, one in the center of each well. The trays are then covered with plastic wrap (Stretch 'n Seal, Colgate Palmolive Company), forming a seal around each

*Supported by PHS grant AI-11717.

well and incubated at room temperature under fluorescent light. Contact between disc and gel is checked at 24 hours and the test is read at 48 hours. In the presence of ADA, ammonia is released from adenosine, changing the pH indicators in the gel from yellow to red. This color change is used as an indicator of ADA activity. The fluorescent light diminishes the brownish discoloration due to hemoglobin, while the plastic wrap limits diffusion of ammonia between wells and prevents the gel from drying out. Control tests are done by omitting adenosine in the gel of some wells, and by using known ADA negative test specimens, such as horse erythrocytes in other wells. The cost of materials is about 1½ cents per sample, and the time required to prepare the reagents and to perform and read the tests is approximately 1 hour for 1 tray. Increased efficiency can be obtained by making up trays prior to use, as trays can be stored satisfactorily for at least three months.

In a first experiment, 34 samples, known to be ADA positive by the method of Kalkar[8] or Hopkinson et al.,[9] were applied using as controls known negative horse red cells or red cells from patients known to have ADAD. In all of the 34 known ADA positive samples, a positive result was obtained on the screening assay, while all known negative specimens were read as negative. In a second experiment, blood spots were obtained from the PKU Laboratory of the New York State Division of Laboratories and Research and plated, randomly intermixed with known ADA negative specimens. When read by two observers unaware of the code, one hundred sixteen of the 118 known negative samples were correctly read while two negatives were read as positive. The latter two samples were run again and were read correctly as negatives. Fifteen hundred and forty blood spots from the 1582 normal subjects were read as ADA positive, while 34 were read as ADA negative. These negative tests were repeated using a second disc cut from the same blood spots and all were then found to be positive. Eight tests could not be interpreted due to heavy fungal contamination of the gel (Table 1).

In further experiments using this method, samples consisting of equal volumes of washed ADA negative horse red cells and known positive human serum showed uniformly negative results. When mixtures of ADA positive and negative erythrocytes were studied, it was found that 15% of red cells in the blood must be ADA positive before even a weak ADA activity could be detected and that a mixture of 25% ADA positive red cells still gave results clearly different from normal.

This method has also been adopted for assaying ADA in substances other than blood, such as serum, tissue homogenates, cultured fibroblasts and column chromotography eluates with pH 6 or less.

The false positive results obtained in 1.7% of cases were apparently caused either by diffusion of ammonia from a neighboring positive well or by con-

TABLE 1

Results of ADA Testing Using 118 Known Negative Samples and 1582
Samples Obtained from the PKU Testing Laboratory

	Known Negative	Normal Subjects
Read Negative	116	34
Read Positive	2	1540

Uninterpretable − 8 (not included in
table).

Accuracy − 97.8%

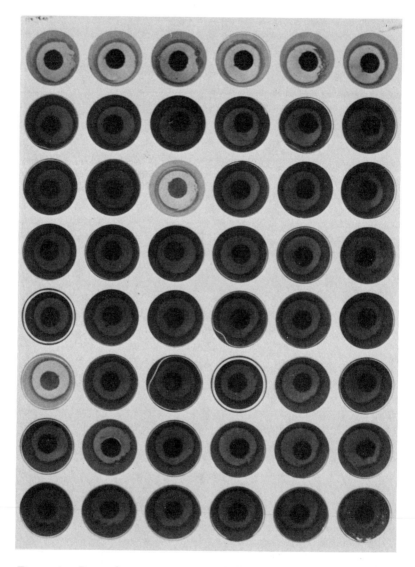

Figure 1. Part of a tray containing 2 blood spots from a known ADA deficient child, with other spots obtained from the PKU testing laboratory. The bottom, control row, does not contain adenosine.

tamination of test materials with alkali. The 2.2% false negative results appeared to be due either to insufficient contact between the blood spots and the gel surface or to as yet inapparent fungal growth on the gel. Negative tests can be readily rechecked by running a second disc from the same blood spot. Persistently negative screening tests should, of course, lead to further analysis for ADA by more quantitative methods.

In screening newborns, two special possible sources of error must be considered. First, it is possible that maternal serum ADA can cross the placenta and be found in the baby's blood. Our experience indicates that this in all likelihood would not give a false positive test in the screening assay. Serum has a low ADA content and, using this method, requires a significantly longer incubation period to become positive. Secondly, a maternal fetal intrauterine red cell transfusion might occur in which the blood from an ADA deficient baby would contain ADA positive red cells. Our studies, however, indicate that a baby with ADAD would have to have in excess of 25% maternal red cells before ADA activity would be detected by this technique.

This method allows screening of newborns for ADA deficiency on a routine basis, particularly in these laboratories where blood spots are already used for the detecting of PKU and other metabolic abnormalities. It should therefore be possible to detect all, or the great majority, of these babies who have CID associated with ADA deficiency. As the frequency of this combination of illnesses is at the present time unknown, the yield of this type of screening is also unknown. Widespread screening of this type will be required before the true frequency of ADA deficiency in the general population can be established. Without this technique, determination of ADA activity in a sufficient number of subjects would take a great amount of time and effort.

A pilot study using this method is at the present time underway at the PKU Laboratory of the New York State Division of Laboratories and Research, New York State Department of Health in Albany, which analyzes blood from all newborns in the eastern half of New York State excepting New York City itself. This study should provide information on the incidence of ADA deficiency in this part of the United States in both normal individuals and in infants with CID and may be of help in determining the usefulness of neonatal screening for ADA.

REFERENCES

1.   E.R. Giblett, J.E. Anderson, F. Cohen, B. Pollara and H.J. Meuwissen, *Lancet II,* 1067, 1972.

2.   J. Dissing and D. Knudsen, *Lancet II,* 1316, 1972.

3. H.J. Meuwissen, R.J. Pickering and B. Pollara, *in* Second International Conference on Primary Immunological Deficiency Disease in Man, R.A. Good and D. Bergsma (Eds.), The National Foundation-March of Dimes, 1974 (in press).

4. B. Pollara, R.J. Pickering and H.J. Meuwissen, *Pediat. Res. 7,* 362, 1973.

5. T. Jenkins, *Lancet 2,* 736, 1973.

6. Workshop Report, This Symposium, p.

7. N. Ressler, *Clin. Chim. Acta 24,* 247, 1969.

8. H.M. Kalkar, *J. Biol. Chem. 167,* 461, 1967.

9. D.A. Hopkinson, P. Cook and H. Harris, *Ann. Hum. Genet. 32,* 361, 1969.

ACKNOWLEDGEMENTS

We thank Miss E. Paolucci and Mr. R. Kaslovsky for their excellent technical assistance, Dr. R. Vanderlinde and Mrs. J. Burns for supplying us with filter-paper blood spots, and Mrs. R. Null for secretarial help.

DISCUSSION

KURT HIRSCHHORN: Dr. Keightley, do you know the sex of the donor of the transplant in your case?

DR. KEIGHTLEY: The donor was found to be a male by the fluorescent Y chromosome technique. Unfortunately, we did not have a difference in sex.

KURT HIRSCHHORN: Are there any tissues from this fetus that you were able to save frozen? I am trying to devise some method, such as lymphocyte stimulation, by which you could detect whether the patient's own lymphocytes are responsive. If you had polymorphic differences of some enzymes, it might be possible to detect a mixture of isozymes. If only the donor's seeded cells respond to PHA or Con-A or whatever the stimulant may be, you would find primarily the donor's isozyme system. I wonder if this is worthwhile looking at from that point of view.

DR. KEIGHTLEY: We attempted to establish a fibroblast line from the fetus but unfortunately it became infected and was lost. We have planned some studies in which we hope to use differential killing of his lymphocytes with host specific and anti-HLA serum, then will examine mitogen responses in the remaining cells.

DR. HADDEN: Dr. Cohen, was there a 2-haplotype difference in each of the mixed leukocyte culture reactions?

DR. COHEN: Yes. The mother was 2, 14, W25 and 17 and the father was W19, W22, 2 and 12. Essentially similar differences existed between other stimulating and responding cells.

DR. HADDEN: It looks, from the ratios of intermixed lymphocyte culture reaction, as though there were low ratios in the interaction that showed the low CML.

DR. COHEN: I don't think that was the case. There was no direct correlation between the ratio of MLC and CML in either the family members or the controls.

DR. HADDEN: I suspect that if you average those ratios of MLC, they would be lower.

BYUNG PARK: Dr. Moore, in your screening effort in newborns have you encountered any ADA negatives?

DR. MOORE: We found two children under screening that are negative and we haven't been able to get blood from them to confirm this finding.

DR. PARK: How many were screened to find these two?

DR. MOORE: The PKU laboratory has been screening for two and a half months. There are several thousand but I don't know exactly how many.

DR. PARK: Could you possibly adapt your methods to detect the carrier?

DR. MOORE: When we were using Petri dishes, I did run Dr. Keightley's child's parents and the child itself, blindly, with just 2 controls and I did manage to pick out the carriers. I don't think it will work on the dispotrays but it is as good as the other method – as a quantitative method.

DWIGHT T. JANERICH (New York State Health Department, Birth Defects Institute, Albany, New York): Dr. Moore, you mention that in preparing for a screening program that you were doing newborn screening. I wonder if any provisions have been made to determine the frequency of ADA in the population which does not result in CID.

DR. MOORE: We screen all newborns. We find ADA deficiency whether it is associated with CID or not. After they are identified we have to find out whether they have disease or not.

RICHARD HONG: If I remember correctly, 7,000 people were tested in Copenhagen and deficiency was found in only two and both of them did, in fact, have CID, so it would appear that it is quite specific. Certainly from the analysis that has come out of this Workshop, only the 12 year old Kalihari bushman is negative and seemed to be normal, so we think it is pretty specific.

J.F. RUDMIN (Clinton County Health Department, Plattsburgh, New York): I am concerned about the normal MLC's in the case of the abnormal CML's in these families. Is it possible that by taking ratios you might have biased the data in one direction? If the responders were low – that is, a low background incorporation themselves – then you wouldn't be able to tell an abnormal response from a low response. It could be that the response would be low. If you just take the amount of incorporation, ignoring the background

— which some people do in interpreting such data — let's say the responders have a low background for one reason or another — if you just take the results without considering the background, is it possible the results would be abnormally low? Is there any evidence by looking at the data that the responder had a low background incorporation?

DR. COHEN: I don't think they were any lower than the unrelated people that we used as controls.

HAROLD LISCHNER (St. Christopher's Hospital for Children, Philadelphia, Pennsylvania): Dr. Cohen, on your chromium assay, what was the range of S values? In other words, the percentage of chromium released in your untreated cells.

DR. COHEN: This usually was in the 20 to 30 percent range as compared to T. More than that and I think you are working on shaky ground. If you have a much higher spontaneous release than that, I don't think the experiment is worth very much.

DR. LISCHNER: What techniques were you using for lymphocyte preparation?

DR. COHEN: These were separated on Ficoll-Hypaque. The lymphocytes and the tests for MLC's were run in microtiter plates.

DR. LISCHNER: Do you have any data on the family members in their family tree who have normal ADA levels?

DR. COHEN: I am beginning to wonder "what is normal?". They had about 2/3 values. The mother's father was a carrier and the father's mother was a carrier. This was borne out further by the serum determinations that Dr. Meuwissen ran on all of these. The father was zero as far as the serum was concerned and the mother was way down in the low range. The other members were all in this low range — in the lower limits of normal — so I really don't know what is normal. At one end of the spectrum is the homogeneous state where you cannot detect ADA and which is associated with marked heterogeneity of expression. It is conceivable that at the other end we might see some minor defects. It might be completely unrelated to ADA but this seems to be the locus that they all have in common and that we have studied in common. So, while it might be very simplistic interpretation at this time, it was very tempting to associate the two things.

ROLLAND WALKER (Rensselaer Polytechnic Institute, Troy, New York): Dr. Keightley, would you please give us "outsiders" some help on that liver transplant? What sort of cell population went into it?

DR. KEIGHTLEY: Really, all the liver was used. The fetus was obtained by hysterotomy. The liver was dissected out, snipped up with scissors and the cells were dispersed by pulling them in and out of a 2½ cc disposable syringe, in a Hank's balanced salt solution supplemented with 10% of the recipient's serum (95% viability by trypan blue exclusion) and the whole lot was given intraperitoneally to the baby at three months of age.

DR. WALKER: What I'm really asking is what kind of cells do you think we're helping?

DR. KEIGHTLEY: I think we've given the patient lymphoid stem cells.

LAUREN PACHMAN: Dr. Keightley, yesterday you presented some data on one phase of platelet agglutination. Was this before the transplantation on the child and were you able to do similar studies on other members of the family?

DR. KEIGHTLEY: The patient (after the transplantation), the mother and the father all seemed to have the same abnormality — defective platelet aggregation.

DR. MEUWISSEN: In determining ADA in lymphocytes, you have to be careful what you do because you are determining ADA in a population consisting of lymphocytes, platelets, granulocytes and monocytes. So you may or may not have ADA in your platelets.

DR. KEIGHTLEY: We haven't established a normal range yet.

DR. GIBLETT: Did I understand you to say that this child was Jk^a negative before and is now about 3 to 7% Jk^a positive?

DR. KEIGHTLEY: Yes.

DR. GIBLETT: You also said there was a question about ADA being present in the red cells.

DR. KEIGHTLEY: We could find no activity before and now find it about 5%.

DR. MEUWISSEN: Could you tell us what the absolute number of white cells is in your child at present and the absolute number of T cells?

DR. KEIGHTLEY: His absolute lymphocyte count is 1000 per cubic millimeter. Approximately 60% form rosettes with sheep cells.

About three months ago he developed a rash. We could find no cellular infiltrate so we really had no good evidence for a graft versus host reaction.

MARY ANN SOUTH (University of Pennsylvania, Philadelphia, Pennsylvania): Did you isolate an Echo virus?

DR. KEIGHTLEY: Initially we got a cytopathic effect on first passage but were unable to isolate anything subsequently.

DR. SOUTH: Clinically, it sounds like a rubeola or rubella-like illness. He had a little fever and a rash and he got over it? Was his spleen enlarged?

DR. KEIGHTLEY: He has not had an enlarged spleen at any time. He was not febrile at the time he had the rash; in fact, he has only been so on two occasions — at one month of age, when he had otitis media before it responded to treatment with ampicillin, then at 71 days post-transplantation when he developed hypertonic dehydration during an episode of diarrhea. His temperature came down when he was rehydrated.

SECTION V

WORKSHOP PARTICIPANTS

Arthur Ammann, San Francisco Medical Center University of California, San Francisco, California

Douglas Biggar, Hospital for Sick Children, Toronto, Canada

Philip Brunell, New York University Medical College, New York, New York

Rebecca Buckley, Duke University, School of Medicine, Durham, North Carolina

Flossie Cohen, Children's Hospital of Michigan, Detroit, Michigan

Valmore F. Cross, St. Peter's Hospital, Albany, New York

Jorgan Dissing, Institute of Forensic Medicine, Copenhagen, Denmark

Eloise Giblett, King County Central Blood Bank, Seattle, Washington

Claude Griscelli, Hospital Necker-Enfants, Paris, France

Rochelle Hirschhorn, New York University Medical Center, New York, New York

Richard Hong, University of Wisconsin, Madison, Wisconsin

Jan Huber, Hospital for Sick Children, Toronto, Canada

Richard Keightley, University of Alabama Hospital, Birmingham, Alabama

John Kersey, University of Minnesota Medical School, Minneapolis, Minnesota

233

J. deKoning, Instituut voor Anthropogenetica, Leiden, Holland

Harold Lischner, St. Christopher's Hospital for Children, Philadelphia, Pennsylvania

W. R. T. Los, Instituut voor Anthropogenetica, Leiden, Holland

Hilaire J. Meuwissen, New York State Health Department, Birth Defects Institute, Albany, New York

Ellen Moore, New York State Health Department, Birth Defects Institute, Albany, New York

Hans Ochs, University of Washington, School of Medicine, Seattle, Washington

Lauren Pachman, Children's Memorial Hospital, Chicago, Illinois

Byung Park, Harbor General Hospital, Torrance, California

Bernard Pollara, New York State Health Department, Kidney Disease Institute, Albany, New York

Fred Rosen, Children's Hospital, Boston, Massachusetts

Donald Singer, Texas Children's Hospital, Houston, Texas

Mary Ann South, University of Pennsylvania, School of Medicine, Philadelphia, Pennsylvania

Diane Wara, San Francisco Medical Center, University of California, San Francisco, California

Justin Wolfson, University of Wisconsin, Madison, Wisconsin

ADA STATUS IN PATIENTS WITH CID

TABLE 1A

Absent Erythrocyte ADA (13 Patients)

Workshop Number	Patient's Initials	Physicians
1	M.K.J.	Dissing, Copenhagen
2	T.H.	Meuwissen and Pollara, Albany
3	J.F.	Ochs, Seattle
37	M.R.	Keightley and Cooper, Birmingham
39	!Kung Boy	Giblett and Jenkins,* Seattle and South Africa
42	P.K.	Los and deKoning, Leiden
53	A.M.	Pickering, Halifax
54	Baby R.	Brunell, New York City
71	K.S.	Cohen, Detroit
80	A.W.	Rosen, Boston
81	W.W.	Rosen
82	J.B.	Rosen
84	J.D.	Park and Higgins, Torrance

*Recent data indicate that some ADA is present in the erythrocytes of this child (T. Jenkins, Personal Communication).

ADA STATUS IN PATIENTS WITH CID

TABLE 1B

Absent or Very Low Serum ADA*

Workshop Number	Patient's Initials	Physicians
9	G. S.	South, Philadelphia
73	F. G.	Singer, Houston
78	C. B.	Hong, Madison

*Serum ADA determinations were done by B. Pollara (See footnote, Table 2C).

TABLE 1C

Low Spleen ADA

Workshop Number	Patient's Initials	Physicians	ADA
57	J. L. O.	Buckley, Durham	0.5% of normal

ADA STATUS IN PATIENTS WITH CID

TABLE 2A

Patients with Erythrocyte ADA (9 Patients)

Workshop Number	Patient's Initials	Physicians	ADA
1-a	K.K. R.J.	Dissing	"normal"
11	D. J. V.	South	1.00*
38	M.P.	Keightley and Cooper	1.00*
48	K.J.	Ammann and Wara	4.0*
51	M.V.	Ammann and Wara	1.19*
52	M. O.	Ammann and Wara	2.79*
59	S.A.	Griscelli, Paris	6.28*
64	C. E. E.	Buckley	"present"
76	T. B.	Hong	1.91*

* μM adenosine deaminated/min/10 ml packed RBC. Values obtained in the laboratory of B. Pollara, Albany. Normal adult values 2.16 $\pm$ 0.65 μM. Little variation (in RBC-ADA values) appears to take place with age. RBC's, maintained under favorable conditions, show little variation in ADA activity. The low ADA values in samples from Workshop Nos. 11, 38 and 51 may have been the result of unfavorable conditions during long transport time.

TABLE 2B

"Normal" Tissue ADA (6 Patients) *

Workshop Number	Patient's Initials	Physicians	ADA
43	Y. D.	Los and deKoning	("Normal" lymphocyte ADA)
44	G. W.	Los and deKoning	("Normal" fibroblast ADA)
55	J. L. S.	Buckley	("Normal" spleen ADA
66	B. M.	Lischner, Philadelphia	("Normal" ADA in many tissues)**
67	T. S.	Lischner	("Normal" ADA in many tissues)**
68	K.S.	Lischner	("Normal" ADA in lung)**

*"Normal" indicates ADA levels in tissues comparable to ADA levels in tissues from patients who did not have CID.

**ADA assay performed in laboratory of H.J. Meuwissen, Albany, New York.

ADA STATUS IN PATIENTS WITH CID

TABLE 2C

Normal Serum ADA* (26 Patients)

Workshop Number	Patient's Initials	Physicians	ADA
4	D.C.	South	1.9
5	D.S.	South	7.9
6	J.K.	South	4.7
8	S.S.	South	2.5
11-a	D.P.V.	South	5.4
12	D.G.	South	3.3
13	T.S.	South	7.8
14	P.Y.	South	8.2
19	R.F.	South	2.4
20	K.R.	Biggar, Minneapolis	Present**
21	L.H.	Biggar	Present**
25	J.W.	Pachman, Chicago	2.5
26	B.H.	Biggar	86.4
27	T.T.	Biggar	1.9
33	C.R.	Biggar	1.8
36	S.S.	Biggar	3.6
56	D.R.R.	Buckley	"Positive"
60	B.O.	Griscelli	10.6
66	B.M.	Lischner	1.4
67	T.S.	Lischner	2.9
68	K.S.	Lischner	0.95
72	K.P.	Singer	10.3
74	J.Q.	Singer	1.9
77	D.C.	Hong	1.0
79	C.P.	Hong	1.6

*Serum values (with the exception of W.S. No. 56) were obtained in the laboratory of B. Pollara, using adenosine fall off method, and are expressed as μM adenosine deaminated/min/L. Normal adult value: 2.70 (range 0.84 − 7.14). For a discussion of the value of serum ADA assays, see Workshop Summary to be published in *J. Pediat.,* February 1975.

**Present on gel assay. Method as presented at the Symposium. (See presentation by E. Moore and H.J. Meuwissen.)

INTRODUCTION TO WORKSHOP PRESENTATIONS

Richard J. Pickering

Advanced planning for the Workshop included the following:

1. Communication with several physicians involved in the care of patients with combined immunological deficiency disorders.

2. These individuals were requested to complete a prepared form which would provide baseline information on each patient. The form was constructed so as to provide clinical, genetic and laboratory information (including adenosine deaminase results), radiological and pathology findings and treatment information. These forms were completed and sent to the coordinator, Dr. Meuwissen, well before the Workshop.

3. It was also requested that x-rays of all patients involved be submitted for study prior to the Workshop. The x-rays were also sent to the coordinator of the Workshop.

4. If tissues were available participants were asked to send representative sections for review.

When all of this information was received by the coordinator, each chart, set of x-rays and tissue sections were given a Workshop number and each patient was subsequently identified by this Workshop number throughout the study period.

Individuals were selected and asked to review all of the submitted data on all the patients prior to the Workshop. The radiologists and the pathologists reviewed their information without any knowledge of the clinical or laboratory findings. Each person was asked to review the patients and submitted material focusing on any features which might serve to separate the patients into sub-groups. The following individuals were asked to review specific areas:

Dr. Flossie Cohen — Clinical Data
Dr. Eloise Giblett — Genetic Data

241

Drs. Arthur Ammann and Diane W. Wara —
Laboratory Data
Drs. Justin Wolfson and Valmore Cross —
Radiology
Drs. Jan Huber and John Kersey — Pathology
Dr. Richard Hong — Treatment
Dr. Bernard Pollara — Methods for Measuring
ADA Activity

When the Workshop convened, it became clear very rapidly that the number of patients was extensive and the nature of their clinical problems diverse. It was decided by concensus that the Workshop would deal first with all patients who showed deficiency or absence of erythrocyte adenosine deaminase. If time permitted, we would then consider patients in whom it had been established that erythrocyte adenosine deaminase was present. Though this latter group was not considered in the Workshop deliberations because of the shortage of time, some of the discussants did include data from this group in their summaries in order to make a comparison between patients with CID, with and without deficiency of erythrocyte adenosine deaminase.

It is the synthesis of these deliberations which will be discussed in the following presentations.

GENETIC ASPECTS

Eloise R. Giblett

Several questions about the genetic aspects of ADA deficiency existed before this Symposium but most of them now seem resolved. First, the autosomal recessive inheritance pattern of ADA deficiency is entirely consistent with homozygosity or "double heterozygosity" at the autosomal structural gene locus for adenosine deaminase. In two families, consanguinity was present, suggesting homozygosity; however, double heterozygosity seems a more likely explanation in those children with unrelated parents.

The likelihood of more than one ADA locus has been quite conclusively laid to rest by Dr. Hirschhorn's studies. The so-called "red cell" form of ADA is partly converted in most tissues to a "storage form", which has a slower electrophoretic mobility. The small amounts of this form of ADA reported to be present in the tissues of some children with ADA deficiency cannot be explained with certainty. Perhaps it reflects instability of the more active form and better stability of the slower component. Another possibility is that the enzyme seen on electrophoresis does not have ADA specificity but can reduce MTT to formazan. This seems unlikely, as does the possibility that the ADA activity belongs to some micro-organisms invading the tissues of these children.

The earlier proposal that the enzyme defect represents a deletion can now be confidently abandoned, both because small amounts of ADA activity were detected in the tissues of some of these children and because the locus for ADA is apparently not on the same chromosome as the HL-A loci.

Finally, since over half of the children reported at the CID Workshop had no evidence of ADA deficiency, it seems highly likely that deficiencies of other enzymes, possibly in the purine, pyrimidine and nucleic acid metabolic pathways, will soon be found to underlie defects in the immune response.

CLINICAL FEATURES

Flossie Cohen

This is a summary of the clinical findings in 23 patients with combined immunodeficiency disease (CID). Erythrocyte adenosine deaminase (ADA) was absent in 12 and normal in 11 other patients. A 12 year old !Kung boy from the Kalahari Desert of Southwest Africa found to lack erythrocyte ADA and described as "healthy" was added to the series, bringing the total of ADA deficient individuals in the list to 13.

There are few if any differences in the clinical presentation or progress between the ADA deficient and the ADA normal patients. CID was manifested before 6 months of age in 22 patients; 1 ADA deficient patient was without symptoms until 2½ years of age while the !Kung boy, also ADA deficient, appears to be healthy at 12 years of age. The preponderance of males in the CID/ADA normal group may be the result of inclusion of patients with the X-linked form of CID since the syndrome of CID and ADA deficiency appears to be an autosomal recessive disorder. Chronic diarrhea and malabsorption, chronic pneumonia and non-infectious skin lesions occurred with equal frequency in both groups. Recurrent otitis media and infections with opportunistic pathogens occurred in both groups though with slightly greater frequency in ADA deficient patients.

Failure to thrive and candidiasis were noted in all cases with CID and absent ADA. By contrast, these clinical problems were present in only 50% of the patients with normal ADA.

The most consistent physical finding in the 2 groups was the absence of tonsils and adenoids in 22 of the 23 patients with CID. Hepatosplenomegaly was less frequent in the group without ADA, occurring only in the 1 patient whose symptoms began at 2½ years of age.

Thus, while there was considerable heterogeneity in the clinical expression of both groups, it was most apparent in the group with absent ADA. At one end of the spectrum, 11 of 13 individuals with no ADA had an onset of symptoms before 6 months of age and died before 2 years of age, while at the other end of the spectrum there is an apparently healthy 12 year old boy. Somewhere in between is a girl, apparently healthy for the first 2½ years of her life before developing symptoms, who subsequently died at 4 years of age.

Clinical Findings and Erythrocyte Adenosine Deaminase (ADA) in 23 Patients
With Combined Immunodeficiency (CID)

| | ADA Present (11)† | ADA Absent (13) | |
		With CID (12)	Without CID* (1)
Sex			
Male	7 (64%)	6 (50%)	1
Female	4 (36%)	7 (58%)	
Onset of Symptoms			
6 Months	11 (100%)	11 (92%)	
6 Months	0 (0%)	1 (8%)	
No symptoms	0 (0%)	0 (0%)	1
Status			
Dead	3 (27%)	5 (42%)	
Alive	8 (73%)	8 (67%)	1
Failure to Thrive	6 (55%)	12 (100%)	
Chronic Diarrhea	4 (36%)	6 (50%)	
Malabsorption	2 (18%)	3 (25%)	
Otitis	4 (36%)	1 (8%)	
Chronic Pneumonia	6 (55)	8 (67%)	
Candidiasis	5 (45%)	12 (100%)	
Opportunistic Pathogens	4 (36%)	9 (75%)	
Non-infectious Skin Lesions	4 (36%)	5 (42%)	
Bone Lesions	0 (0%)	4 (33%)	
Palpable Lymph Nodes	2 (18%)	1 (8%)	
"Absent" Tonsils & Adenoids	10 (90%)	12 (100%)	
Splenomegaly	2 (18%)	1 (8%)	
Hepatomegaly	3 (27%)	1 (8%)	

†This table includes W.S. No. 15; this patient was not included in the summary published in the Journal of Pediatrics because her ADA data were lacking.

*!Kung Boy

LABORATORY DATA

D.W. Wara
A.J. Ammann

In reviewing the patients' laboratory data and attempting to define their immunodeficiency disorders we were confronted with numerous problems. The term "combined immunodeficiency" (CID) describes patients with defective antibody and cell mediated immunity. Well characterized immunodeficiency syndromes such as ataxia telangiectasia, Wiskott-Aldrich syndrome and DiGeorge syndrome could be included under the term CID but because they have established associated defects they have been separately categorized.

Patients with RBC adenosine deaminase (ADA) deficiency, who were under primary consideration in this Symposium, had varying degrees of antibody and cellular immunodeficiency. We deliberately chose rigid criteria to define absence of antibody or cell mediated immunity. Patients were placed in the category of severe CID if all parameters of both antibody and cell mediated immunity studied were abnormal.

Evaluation of Antibody Mediated Immunity

Quantitative immunoglobulins: All five classes (IgG, IgM, IgA, IgD and IgE) should be measured. However, the majority of patients studied had only IgG, IgM and IgA quantitated.

Antibody response following immunization: Ideally, all patients should have been challenged with both a protein and a polysaccharide antigen. Evidence suggests that there may be thymic dependence and independence, respectively.[1] Additional information could have been obtained utilizing other immunogens but the hazards involved would have outweighed the possible information derived. Typhoid immunization has resulted in severe systemic reactions when given to some immunodeficient children.[2] Live virus should never be administered to patients suspected of having immunodeficiency as this has not only resulted in progressive vaccinia with smallpox vaccination[3] but also paralytic polio following oral polio immunization.[4]

Peripheral blood B cells: Newer methodology has permitted the specific identification of peripheral blood lymphocytes as either T or B cells. B cells

247

comprise approximately 25 to 30 percent of peripheral lymphocytes.[5] Fluorescein labeled anti-IgG, IgM and IgA has been used to identify lymphocytes bearing specific surface immunoglobulin or immunoglobulin-like receptors. A second method utilizes the rosette technique to identify peripheral B lymphocytes in their binding affinity for antibody and complement coated sheep red blood cells (EAC rosettes).[6] The percentage of peripheral B lymphocytes determined by both methods correlates well.

Additional criteria for antibody mediated immunity: The presence or absence of isohemagglutinins, lymph node morphology and intestinal histology are insufficiently precise to aid in classification. However, the absence of plasma cells may be an additional criteria for the diagnosis of severe CID.

Evaluation of Cell Mediated Immunity

Cell mediated immunity has only recently been assayed precisely. Certain well established procedures are helpful but their limitations must be recognized.

Delayed hypersensitivity: Skin tests are frequently negative in children and are only of definite value when they are nonreactive following a previously documented immunization or infection. In our experience, the most useful skin test antigen is *Candida* because of frequent exposure to this agent. Positive reactions to delayed hypersensitivity skin tests generally indicate intact cellular immunity; however, an Arthrus reaction may be confused with specific delayed hypersensitivity if the lesion has not been observed as a continuum. Deliberate sensitization to chemicals such as dinitrochlorobenzene (DNCB) may likewise produce reactions which are difficult to interpret. The solutions are frequently made up in acetone and are susceptible to changes induced by light and evaporation. A challenge dose may occasionally become a re-sensitizing dose.

Mitogen stimulation of lymphocytes in vitro: Phytohemagglutinin (PHA) is considered a potent mitogen primarily of T cells. Ideally, multiple doses of PHA and normal controls should be included in each study. The interpretation of results should be based on all data (resting counts, stimulated counts and stimulation index). Other mitogens such as Concanavalin A and pokeweed are not clearly stimulators of primarily T cells. They are therefore not included as studies used to establish a diagnosis.

Response to allogeneic cells: The ability of T cells to recognize foreign cells can be measured by the mixed lymphocyte culture response (MLC). Although some patients with severe CID have been reported to have a positive MLC response, this appears to be rare.

T cell rosettes: The ability of isolated peripheral blood lymphocytes to form rosettes with uncoated sheep red blood cells identified 60-70% as T cells in the normal population.[7] Patients with severe CID probably have values of less than 10%.

Classification of Patients Based on Laboratory Data

The patients presented to the Symposium were documented as having normal, decreased or increased circulating B cells, lymphocyte response to PHA and in MLC, and T cell rosettes; unfortunately, exact data were not available for interpretation. As selective deficiencies of T cell function exist, patients were classified as severe CID only if they were deficient in all parameters tested: absent or decreased IgG, IgM and IgA, absent antibody response to immunogens, absent or decreased circulating B cells as determined by fluorescent studies or EAC rosettes, absent delayed hypersensitivity skin tests, absent or decreased lymphocyte response to PHA and MLC and decreased T cell rosettes. Patients with residual B cell immunity or minimal evidence of functioning cellular immunity were classified as variable CID. It is important to note that the majority of patients reviewed during the Symposium had been studied immunologically at only one point in time and not sequentially. Immunological attrition may occur in a subpopulation of these patients and their classification as variable CID rather than severe CID may only reflect the time at which they were studied.

Twelve of the 22 patients studied immunologically had absent RBC ADA. Eight of the twelve patients with absent RBC ADA were classified as severe CID (Table 1). In this group, one ADA positive and one ADA negative patient had minimal lymphocyte response in MLC. There was no other evidence of immunological activity. Seven of the eight patients with severe CID and absent RBC ADA had x-ray findings described by J. Wolfson as pseudo-achondroplasia. The eighth patient had cupping and flaring or anterior rib ends. None of the three patients described with normal RBC ADA and severe CID had bony radiological abnormalities.

Four of the 12 patients with absent RBC ADA were classified as variable CID (Table 2). None of the four had the radiological findings present in patients with severe CID and absent RBC ADA. One of the four patients with variable CID (W.S. No. 2) had documented loss of both antibody and cellular immunity over time (immunological attrition). The seven patients with present RBC ADA who were classified as variable CID were indistinguishable immunologically from those with absent RBC ADA.

An additional patient with absent RBC ADA, a !Kung boy from the Kalahari desert, is not included in the tables because of inadequate data available. He had normal quantitative immunoglobulins, normal numbers of circulating lymphocytes and a weak response to tuberculin skin test; no *in vitro* lymphocyte function tests were performed. He would most likely be classified as a normal child or as variable CID.

In summary, a review of available data in patients with immunodeficiency with and without RBC ADA deficiency reveals one distinctive group. In this group there is absence of RBC ADA and severe deficiency of antibody and cell mediated immunity. Later, this group was noted to have characteristic radiologic abnormalities. The remainder of patients with RBC ADA absence did not appear to be distinguishable from patients with identical immunologic abnormalities and presence of RBC ADA.

REFERENCES

1. D. Amerding and D.H. Katz, *J. Exp. Med. 139,* 24, 1974.

2. A.J. Ammann and D.W. Wara, *in* Cellular Immunodeficiency Disorders in Infants and Children, E.R. Stiehm and V.A. Fulginiti (Eds.). W.B. Saunders Co., Philadelphia, p. 236, 1973.

3. V.A. Fulginiti, H.C. Kempe, W.E. Hathaway, D.S. Pearlman, O.F. Suber, J.J. Eller, J.J. Joyner and A. Robinson, *in* Birth Defects, Immunologic Deficiency Diseases in Man, Vol. IV, No. 1, p. 129, February, 1968.

4. F.D. Feigin, M.A. Guggenheim and S.D. Johnson, *Pediatrics 370,* 630, 1966.

5. H.M. Grey, E. Rabellino and B. Pirofsky, *J. Clin. Invest. 50,* 2268, 1971.

6. E.M. Sherach, R. Herberman and M.M. Frank, *J. Clin. Invest. 51,* 1933, 1972.

7. R.C. Williams, J.R. DeBoard, O.J. Mellbye, R.P. Messner and F.D. Lindstron, *J. Clin. Invest. 52,* 283, 1973.

TABLE 1
Immunological Data in Patients with "Severe" CID
(Group I)

W.S. No.	IgG	IgM	IgA	Antibody Production	Circulating B cells	PHA	MLC Response	T cell Rosettes
ADA Negative								
1	<200	10	0	0	ND	0	0	ND
3	134	15	0	0	ND	0	ND	ND
42	→	0	0	ND	ND	0	ND	ND
37	Maternal	0	0	ND	ND	0	ND	0
53	70	0	0	ND	ND	0	0	0
54	310	0	0	ND	10%	0	→	0
82	Maternal	0	0	0	ND	0	0	ND
84	230	0	0	ND	ND	0	0	ND
ADA Positive								
15*	70	0	0	0	ND	0	→	ND
52	175	8	0	0	ND	0	0	ND
1-a	<25mg %	<10mg %	<10mg %	0	ND	0	0	ND

*In the summary prepared for the Journal of Pediatrics this patient was omitted because her ADA data were lacking.

251

TABLE 2
Immunological Data in Patients with "Less Severe" CID
(Group II)

W.S. No.	IgG	IgM	IgA	Antibody Production	Circulating B cells	PHA	MLC Response	T cell Rosettes
ADA Negative								
2	1600→200	600→20	70	Variable	ND	0-→	0-→	→
81	Maternal	0	0	ND	0	↓ 5-15x	→	→
71	600-1800	100-1300	80	+	Normal	→	→	Normal
80	540	75	50	0	ND	0	0	ND
ADA Positive								
11	0	0	0	0	←→	0	0	→
38	1300	11	0	ND	→	0	0	→
48	11	340	0	0	ND	0	0	→
51	2500	205	86→	0	←	→	0	→
59	↓	N		0	N	0	N	0
64	145	18	10	0	N	0	0	→
76	1160	50	970	+	N	0	0	→

DISCUSSION

DR. WARA: There is one patient who is considered in the ADA positive group who is 15 years old and was variable in deficiency. There was no one who even approached that age in the ADA negative, severe CID group.

DR. ROSEN: I just wanted to make the comment that what is emerging is recommendations for the study of these patients. The WHO committee on primary immunodeficiency has considered at great length the work-up of patients with primary immune deficiency and part of this consideration is what antigens should be used to study antibody formation, etc. Two principles emerged from a rather lengthy discussion: (1) not to use any live antigens — with the single exception of ΦX 174, which the Seattle group has proved extremely useful in detecting certain subgroups of immunodeficiency and (2) to use antigens that are useful in protecting the patient. For that reason immunization with KLH was carefully considered and was discarded as a recommended procedure.

THE RADIOGRAPHIC FINDINGS IN FORTY-NINE PATIENTS WITH COMBINED IMMUNODEFICIENCY

Justin J. Wolfson
Valmore F. Cross

INTRODUCTION

We examined the radiographs of 49 patients with combined immuno-deficiency disease. Type and number of studies available were exceedingly variable. The name of the patient, his institution and history number and other identifying marks were covered with opaque tape and all films and film jackets were coded. All clinical data, except for dates of birth and of examination, were intentionally withheld from us.

All films were studied by each of the authors independently and then together. The findings on each film were annotated. The lungs were evaluated according to the radiographic criteria previously developed by one of us for a group of patients who had either hypogammaglobulinemia or combined immunodeficiency disease.[1]

Until shortly before our presentation to the Workshop we did not know what the erythrocyte ADA status was for the 49 patients on whom we had one or more films. As it turns out, 13 of these 49 have an absence of erythrocyte ADA.

When we then related the ADA status with the disease categories we had determined (Chart 1) we found that every patient with bone abnormalities lacked erythrocyte ADA. On the basis of this new knowledge, we then critically reviewed our data and our films and discovered 3 or 4 additional patients with bone abnormalities. All of these data are summarized in Chart 1.

THYMUS

All of our patients have marked reduction in size, or apparent absence

255

of, the thymus. We evaluated the anterior mediastinum both in frontal and in lateral projections. Although the anterior mediastinum is narrower than normal in the frontal projection,* the appearance is variable and therefore much less helpful than in the lateral view.

In the normal infant or small child (Fig. 1A) the retrosternal lung is only hazily radiolucent and merges almost imperceptibly with the more opaque cardiac silhouette and proximal great vessels. In virtually all of the 47 patients on whom adequate lateral films were available, the anterior margins of soft tissue structure, i.e., of the heart and great vessels, are sharply demarcated against the black or hyperlucent retrosternal lung lying in front of them (Fig. 1B). In none of these is there evidence of a soft tissue "mass" lesion within, or silhouetted against, the zone of hyperlucent lung to suggest the presence of thymic tissue. Lateral body section radiographs of the thymic area are not available on any of these patients. This technique might possibly have delineated rudimentary thymic tissue not visible on plain films.

LUNG

Bronchopneumonia is evident in 27 patients and changes suggestive of or consistent with *Pneumocystis carinii* pneumonia in 7. Four show air trapping and 5 atelectasis.

Unequivocal or probable thickening of the walls of major bronchi ("tram" lines) is present in 29 patients (Fig. 2C). Of special interest are 13 who showed generalized prominence of small linear markings throughout the lungs (Fig. 2A and B).

Of the 13 patients in whom we recorded these findings, 9 are ADA negative and of these 9, 5 have the unusual bone changes to be described below. The ages of the patients at the time these lung changes were manifest varied from 4 through 18 months. Average age was 12.6 months.

MISCELLANEOUS FINDINGS

The 10 patients on whom satisfactory films of the neck are available show markedly diminished or apparently absent adenoidal tissue. Only 2 of the 10 are less than 6 months of age and the average of the group is 9.2 months. One patient shows substantial enlargement of the mediastinal and hilar nodes. One patient shows evidence of cardiac failure and 2 of his siblings, also with CID,

---

*Two patients, W.S. No. 59 and 71, had normal thymic shadows on early radiographs of the chest. At age 3 years No. 71 developed CID at which time her chest film showed an absence of the thymus.

256

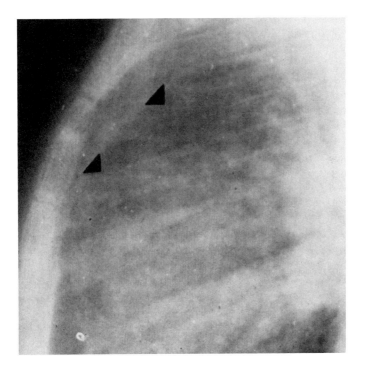

Fig. 1A and 1B.   On the left (1A), a lateral view of a normal infant does not permit delineation of soft tissue structures (arrows) behind the sternum. On the right, however, (1B) which is a lateral view of an infant with CID, the anterior heart border and great vessels are sharply defined (arrows) because of the absence of the thymus.

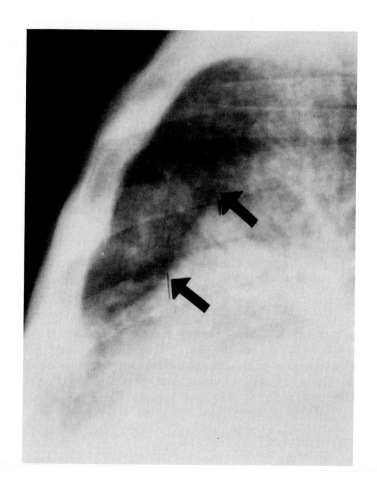

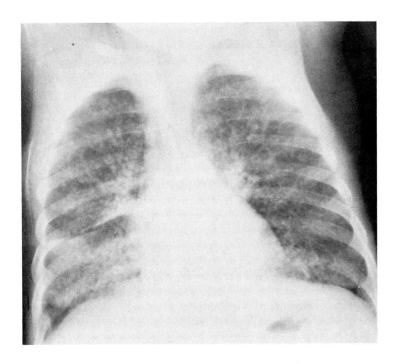

Fig. 2A, 2B, 2C, 2D and 2E. Fig. 2A is that of a patient with CID and ADA positive erythrocytes. Fig. 2B–E are of another patient, also with CID and ADA positive erythrocytes. In 2A and 2B the mediastinum (arrows) is narrow because the thymus is small to absent; in both, a "thicket" produced by superimposition of branching white lines is distributed through both lung fields. Fig. 2C is a magnified view of the left lung shown in 2B. Fig. 2D a view of the same patient on a separate occasion, shows less disease than do 2B and 2C but it does demonstrate well several long, thick, straight, radially oriented white lines at the left base which are the "tram" lines of thickened bronchial walls. Fig. 2E (far right) is a microscopic section of the lung on the same patient secured at postmortem. The respiratory bronchiole shown is markedly thickened by inflammation and fibrosis. Histologic study suggests that the "thicket" pattern in the lungs of CID patients is due to thickening of the walls of small bronchi and bronchioli.

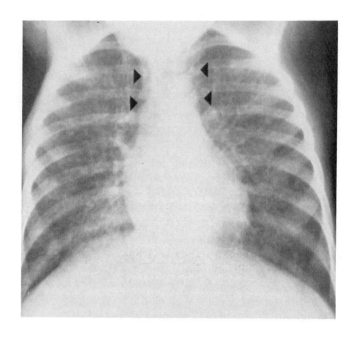

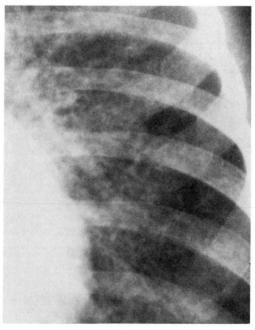

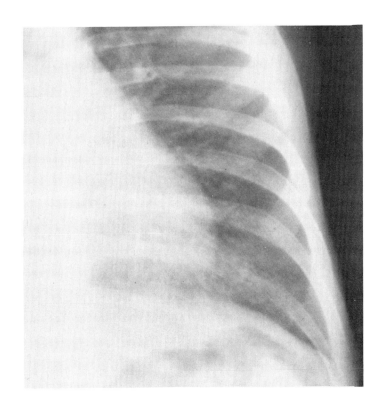

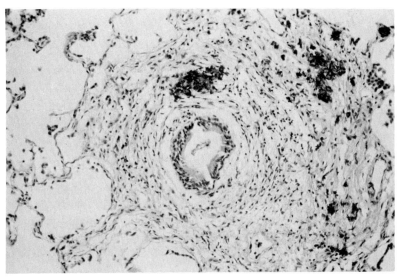

have an apparent enlargement of the heart with normal vascularity of the lung fields. One patient has pleural effusion as well as anasarca, ascites and edema of the small intestine. Six patients have thickening of the valvulae conniventes and/or widening of the lumen of the small intestine.

BONE CHANGES

Perhaps our most important observations as they relate to the purpose of this Workshop and Symposium are a constellation of bony abnormalities which we found exclusively in our ADA negative patients.

Concavity and Flaring of Ribs

Concavity or prominent cupping of the anterior ends of the ribs, in association with flaring, is present in 9 patients (Fig. 3).* All but 2 have absence of erythrocyte ADA. These 2 (W.S. No. 9 and No. 78) have an absence of serum ADA but have no erythrocyte ADA determinations.

Structural detail of the ends of the anterior ribs is best delineated in oblique and lateral positions and frequently obscured or inapparent in a frontal view. Since we frequently had available only frontal views, we may have missed one or more patients with such abnormalities.

Pelvis

Of the 9 patients who have concavity and flaring of their anterior ribs, 5 show moderate to severe abnormality of their pelves. On 3 of the other 4 (W.S. No. 9, No. 57 and No. 84), we have no pelvic films.** The fourth (W.S. No. 78) has an apparently normal pelvis.***

The pelves of these 5 patients (Fig. 4) are vertically short and their width/height ratios correspondingly increased. Their ilia are "squared off", though with slight flare. This appearance is enhanced by a "low-set" sacrum, shortening of the lower portion of the ilium and a broad horizontal

---

*A report of one of these patients has been published recently by Yount et al.[2] An oblique radiograph of the rib cage, in their Fig. 1, demonstrated the rib abnormality beautifully and unequivocally.

**W.S. No. 9 has ADA negative serum but no RBC determination. W.S. No. 57 has ADA negative spleen and thymus but no RBC determination. W.S. No 84 has ADA negative RBC's.

***W.S. No. 78 is the only known patient with abnormal anterior ribs to have a normal pelvis. She has an absence of ADA in her serum but had no red blood cell ADA determination. In addition to CID, she was known to have the Wiedemann-Beckwith syndrome.

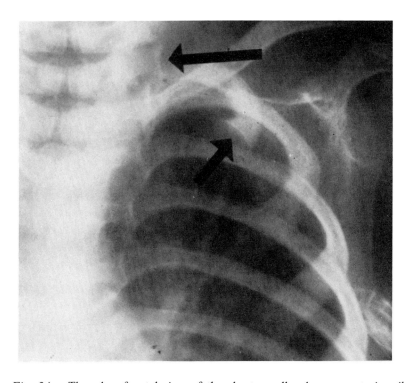

Fig. 3A. Though a frontal view of the chest usually obscures anterior rib detail, flaring and concavity of the first rib (short arrow) are well demonstrated. Upper transverse processes (long arrows) also are concave and flared where they articulate with posterior ribs. In other patients (see text) the margins of these bones are straight and separated by a slight radiolucent gap, such that the vertical sequence of these gaps presents, to the eye, as a long radiolucent band. Incidental finding is a broader-than-average cleft between the two halves of the vertebral arch.

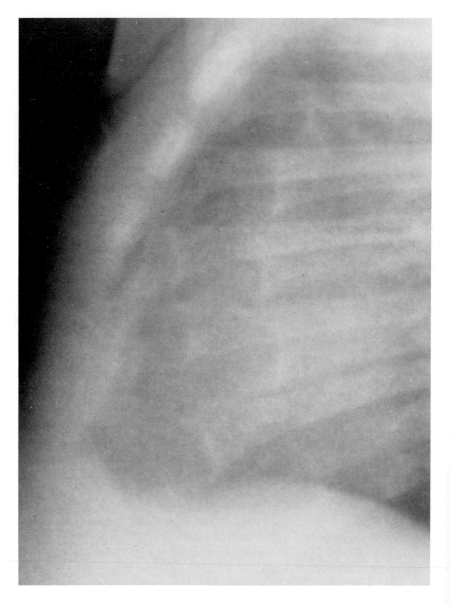

Fig. 3B. Lateral chest on W.S. No. 3, a patient with absence of RBC ADA. Anterior ribs are concave and flared but less so than in some of our patients. The pelvic configuration of this patient (Fig. 4B) is subtly but clearly abnormal. (Courtesy of H. Ochs, M.D. and R.J. Wedgwood, M.D.)

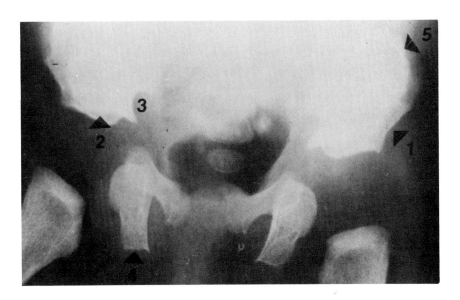

Fig. 4A (left) and 4B (center) are pelves of infants with red cell ADA deficiency. Fig. 4C (right) is a normal pelvis for comparison. The pelves in Fig. 4A, which is an example of severe configurational change and Fig. 4B, which is an example of minimal change, are clearly structurally different from the pelvis in Fig. 4C (right) which is normal.

Width/height ratio and the size of the cartilaginous areas are increased in Fig. 4A and 4B, as compared with 4C. In addition, though variably in 4A and 4B, the ilia are "squared off",[1] acetabular roofs are flat and long,[2] the lower ilia and sacrosciatic notches are short,[3] ischia are squat and untapered,[4] and growth arrest lines (only in Fig. 4A) are unusually thick.[5] (Courtesy of R. Pickering, M.D. (Fig. 4A), and H. Ochs, M.D. and R.J. Wedgwood, M.D. (Fig. 4B).

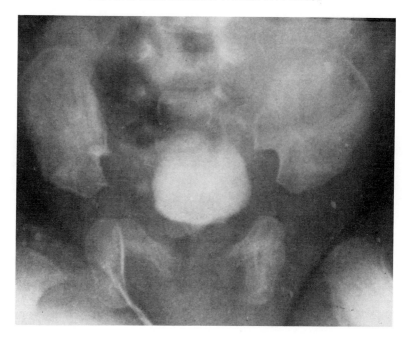

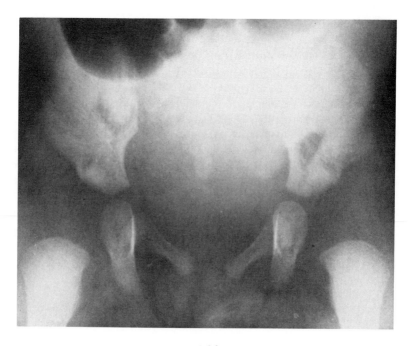

acetabulum. The sacrosciatic notches, though variable in size, are correspondingly small. The ischia are broad, vertically disposed and squat, terminating abruptly with straight or concave margins and often with small, medial cortical spurs.

Transverse Process-Rib Articulation

An additional finding relates to the posterior rib cage (Fig. 3A). Normally the proximal portions of the ribs and the transverse processes of the vertebrae are slightly convex at their ends and overlap in frontal view. In 5 patients, all with an absence of ADA, the following variations are noted: transverse processes are short and, for the most part, do not overlap the ends of the ribs. The edges of each are vertically straight or concave rather than convex so that, to the eye, the series of vertical gaps between each two bones appears as a continuous, radiolucent stripe or band on either side of the midline. The demonstration of this finding requires good positioning. Also, it is quite variable and may be seen occasionally in normal infants.

Vertebrae

Slight decrease in height, or platyspondyly, of thoracic and lumbar vertebrae, with corresponding increase in width of the interspaces, is clearly evident in 4 patients with an absence of erythrocyte-ADA. In 2 of the 4, a slight kyphos and anterior beaking are present at the L1-L2 and L2-L5 levels, respectively. Interpediculate distances in 2 bone-affected patients, 2 and 4 months of age respectively, show an increase from L1 through L5 of 1 to 1.5 millimeters. This is in contrast to infantile achondroplasia in which lumbar interpediculate distances remain the same or decrease.[3]

Growth Arrest Lines

Growth arrest lines, or strata, are in essence an indelible imprint of metabolic insult. They are non-specific, commonly present in otherwise normal children and invariably thin. We saw these lines in at least 6 patients, 3 of whom have an absence of erythrocyte ADA. At least 2 of these 3 manifest uniquely thick growth arrest lines, most conspicuous in the ilia (Fig. 5).

Trabecular Paucity

Two or our patients, both with an absence of erythrocyte ADA, demonstrate hyperlucency at the ends of their long bones. As with growth arrest lines, trabecular paucity, or "trabecular poverty" as it has been called by Park, is a nonspecific finding, its pathogenesis probably being related to nutritional and/or metabolic aberration.[4]

267

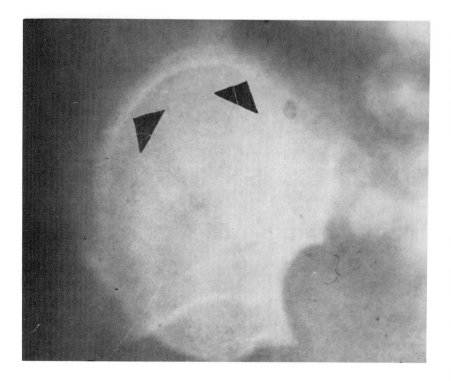

Fig. 5A and 5B. Thick, opaque growth arrest lines (sometimes called bands or strata): (5A) in the ilium and (5B) in the right humerus (arrows). Growth arrest lines, which probably result from nutritional or metabolic disturbance, are common and invariably are thin. Rarely are they broad as here. Their unique thickness in our patients, in association with CID and red cell ADA deficiency, probably is related to immaturity of cartilage cells in the growth plate (see text).

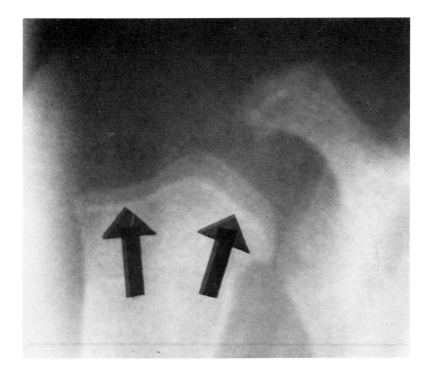

EXTREMITIES

In all patients the bones of the arms and thighs (humeri and femurs) are longer than the bones of the respective forearms and legs. On the basis of tables provided by Maresh,[5] arm-forearm and femur-leg ratios are normal. However, overall extremity lengths are very short — below the tenth percentile in 1 measured patient. Occasional metaphyses in some of the ADA negative patients are slightly irregular.

Osteoporosis, manifested as thinning of cortex and hyperlucency, is common and striking in at least 8 both ADA positive and negative patients.

Bone age as determined from sparse hand films and the appearance of the proximal humeral epiphyses is slightly reduced in our CID patients.

DISCUSSION

Perhaps the best known radiographic sign of immunodeficiency disease is hypoplasia or apparent absence of adenoidal tissue. This is evident in every patient on whom films are available, 10 in all. The average age of this group is 9.2 months. While absence of an adenoidal shadow in children over 6 months of age should suggest immunodeficiency, its absence in normal children younger than that is frequent.[6] This examination then should be reserved primarily for children older than 6 months and should be considered part of a thorough patient workup.

The chest examination fulfills several diagnostic functions in patients with CID. First of all, a sharply defined retrosternal hyperlucency, evident in a lateral view, is presumptive evidence of thymic absence. *Pneumocystis carinii* pneumonia generally presents an appearance sufficiently characteristic, especially if related with clinical findings, to be diagnostic. However, immediate additional diagnostic studies for its positive identification may well be required. "Tram" lines (Fig. 2C), while evident under various circumstances in some children — notably those with asthma, cystic fibrosis, bronchiectasis and intercurrent infection — are common also in hypogammaglobulinemia and CID.[1] Uniquely characteristic of CID, however, is the prominent, symmetric, often thicket-like branching linear pattern in the lungs of these patients (Fig. 2).[1] There is clinical and histological evidence to suggest that this appearance is due to inflammatory and/or fibrous thickening of the walls of small bronchi, terminal bronchioli and even respiratory bronchioli (Fig. 2D).[7]

However valuable these radiographic observations may be, it is not these but rather the several bony aberrations which characterize certain of the ADA negative patients, which have fired the interest and concern of our Workshop and Symposium participants.

270

Several reports of bony abnormalities in association with CID are available. Davis[8,9] appears to have been the first to recognize that the bony changes, though in some respects resembling those of achondroplasia, differ significantly from the latter and that together with CID they constitute a new "syndrome".

For our purposes 2 papers are particularly helpful since they include radiographs and descriptions.[10,11] In fact, the 2 patients with "thymic alymphoplasia" reported by Alexander and Dunbar[10] appear to have exactly the same radiographic manifestations as do ours. We believe that they, too, must have had an absence of erythrocyte ADA.

A discussion of radiographic differential diagnoses for our patients is beyond the scope of this paper. Good discussions of achondroplasia[3,12] and other causes of short-limbed dwarfism with which our patients might be confused[13,14] are available.

Concavity and flaring of anterior rib margins are not specific for ADA deficiency CID. They are present in rickets as well as in a number of other syndromes.[14] However, the sign is valuable in its own right and deserves wider recognition. It is picked up with ease — all that is required are PA and lateral chest films — and, in the bargain, other areas may be checked out at the same time: the anterior mediastinum for absence of thymus, the lungs for infection and bronchiolar wall thickening, the posterior rib articulations for diminished overlap and the spine for platyspondyly.

One of the 9 patients with anterior rib changes deserves special comment; this is a patient of Dr. Rosen's. A film at 3 months showed marked cupping and flaring of ribs. At 9 months, after successful therapy of his CID, the cupping and flaring had resolved almost completely. Another who had received no therapy still had prominent cupping and flaring at 7 months. We therefore suggest that regression of these findings may be due to normalization of cartilage formation after treatment.

Although the bones in such syndromes as achondroplasia, chondroectodermal dysplasia, asphyxiating thoracic dystrophy, thanatophoric dwarfism, as well as in our CID-ADA negative patients, resemble one another in certain configurational respects, these syndromes are readily distinguishable. It is likely that the specific pattern of bone development in each of these conditions is genetically "programmed" into individual epiphyseal plates.

Histological changes of the growth plate, or physeal cartilage, in some of these conditions have been described.[15,16] Most recently, Rimoin[17] has made efforts to classify short-limbed dwarfism on the basis of specific histologic features of chondro-osseous junctions.

In the case reports of their 2 patients, Alexander and Dunbar[10] have included the histologic descriptions of the chondro-osseous junctions. In both instances, the cartilage was characterized by an absence of columnization, an overall thinness and a paucity and immaturity of chondroblasts. Although the histologic appearance of the growth plates of our patients is not known as of this writing, we believe that it is probably identical to that noted by Alexander and Dunbar for their patients. Specific generalized growth aberrations due to abnormalities of physeal cartilage frequently are most prominent at the sites of most rapid growth. The anterior rib ends are the fastest growing of all bones in the infant[4] and might therefore be expected to manifest the most florid alterations.

While it is possible that disordered column formation may contribute to widening of the chondro-osseous junction and, as with rickets, help produce the phenomenon of flaring, Rimoin explains the concavity and flaring ("cupping") differently. He thinks it is due to periosteal bony overgrowth ("cuffing") of the non-ossified perichondrium which surrounds the epiphyseal plate.[17]

The histologic findings reported by Alexander and Dunbar and the phenomenon of cuffing may help explain the decreased growth rate and unusual contours we have described — specifically the diminished overlap of transverse processes and posterior ribs, platyspondyly and shortening of the ischia without distal tapering. Other configurational changes, as in the ilia, are more complex and subtle than these but they, too, probably are a culmination of the same pathogenetic mechanisms.

This thesis is supported by the presence both in our patients and, as gleaned through inspection of published radiographs, in Alexander and Dunbar's patients, of thick growth arrest lines. Since thin growth arrest lines, or strata, are usual and thick lines are rare,[18] the occurrence of thick lines in these patients requires explanation.

Since the thickness of the growth arrest line, or stratum, is proportionate to the length of time required for cartilage cells to mature, which is the "recovery" period,[4] the presence of thick lines in our patients as well as in those reported by Alexander and Dunbar, presumes a diminished growth rate of the bones. Therefore the thickened strata are a reflection of a basic immaturity of growth plate chondroblasts.

In "the present state of the art" our concepts of short-limbed dwarfism are descriptively and visually derived. The radiograph has served us well as a means of distinguishing a variety of phenotypic expressions. However, it is to be hoped that our overall knowledge of short-limbed dwarfism will be enhanced as pathogenetic mechanisms are better understood.

Radiographic abnormalities are tabulated on 49 patients with CID, 13 of whom have an absence of erythrocyte ADA. The correlation of radiographic and ADA data provides a means of distinguishing 2 categories of radiographic findings: (1) those applicable to all patients with CID and (2) those applicable only to patients with ADA-deficient CID.

In the first category are (1) osteoporosis, (2) a unique and characteristic lung pattern and (3) a small or absent thymus gland.

In the second category are 9 patients who manifest, in addition, one or more of the following bone abnormalities:

1. Cupping and flaring of the anterior rib ends.
2. Broad, vertically short pelvis, relatively square ilia and short, bluntly-ending ischia.
3. Alteration of contour and articulation of transverse processes and posterior ribs.
4. Platyspondyly.
5. Abnormally thick growth arrest lines.

Explanations for these radiographic findings are suggested.

ACKNOWLEDGEMENTS

With gratitude, the authors express their appreciation to Dr. John Opitz for his review of this manuscript and for his helpful comments.

REFERENCES

1. J.J. Wolfson, Presentation before the Twelfth Annual Meeting of the Society for Pediatric Radiology, Washington, D.C., September 29, 1969.

2. J. Yount, P. Nichols *et al., J. Pediat. 84,* 173, 1974.

3. L.O. Langer, P. A. Bauman *et al., Am. J. Roentgenol. 100,* 12, 1967.

4. E.A. Park, *Pediatrics (Supplement) 33,* 815, 1964.

5. M.M. Maresh, *in* Human Growth and Development, R.W. McCannon, (Ed.), Charles C. Thomas,Springfield, Illinois, p. 155, 1970.

6. M.A. Capitanio and J.A. Kirkpatric, *Radiology 96,* 389, 1970.

7. J.J. Wolfson, Personal communication.

8. J.A. Davis, *Brit. Med. J. 2,* 1371, 1966.

9. J.A. Davis, *Brit. Med. J. 3,* 110, 1967.

10. W.J. Alexander and J.S. Dunbar, *Ann. Radiol. (Paris) 11,* 389, 1968.

11. R.A. Gatti, N. Platt *et al., J. Pediat. 75,* 675, 1969.

12. F.N. Silverman, *in* Progress in Pediatric Radiology. Intrinsic Diseases of Bones, H.J. Kaufmann (Ed.), S. Karger, Basel, Volume 4, p. 94, 1973.

13. H.J. Kaufmann (Ed.), Progress in Pediatric Radiology. Intrinsic Diseases of Bones, Volume 4, S. Karger, Basel, 1973.

14. R.M. Saldino, *Med. Radiogr. Photogr. 61,* 49, 1973.

15. C.E. Anderson, T.C. Jackson *et al., J. Bone Joint Surg. 44A1,* 295, 1962.

16. I.V. Ponseti, *J. Bone Joint Surg. 52,* 701, 1970.

17. D.L. Rimoin, *in* Progress in Pediatric Radiology. Intrinsic Diseases of Bones, H.J. Kaufmann (Ed.), S. Karger, Basel, Volume 4, p. 68, 1973.

18. J.J. Wolfson and R.R. Engel, *Radiology 92,* 1055, 1969.

RESUME OF RADIOGRAPHIC DATA ON 49 PATIENTS WITH CID*
(Italicized numbers indicate patients with absent red cell ADA)

		(A) ADA RBC NEG + ADA RBC POS	(B) ADA RBC NEG ONLY
NUMBERS OF PATIENTS**			
I.	Total number of patients	49	
II.	Total number with at least one chest film	46	
III.	Total number with absent red cell ADA		13
THYMUS			
IV.	Absence of thymus W.S. *1*, 1A, *2*, 5, *9,* 12, 25, *37,* *42*, 43, 46, 47, 52, *53,* 55, 59, 64, 65, 69, 70, 71, 76, *81*	23	7
V.	Normal thymus W.S. 59A, 71	2	0
LUNG			
VI.	Pneumonia W.S. *2, 3,* 4, 5, *6, 9,* 19, 20, 25	27	9

*Of the patients with bony aberrations, three had no ADA determinations of their RBC's: W.S. No. 9, 57 and 78. Each had absence of ADA by other determinations, however:

W.S. No. 9 — absence of ADA in the serum.

W.S. No. 57 — absence of ADA in thymus and spleen.

W.S. No. 78 — absence of ADA in the serum.

Each of these is underlined in Chart I and has been included in the tabulation of "ADA RBC NEG ONLY".

**12 ADA positive patients included in these tables were not included in the Workshop summary prepared for the Journal of Pediatrics because of insufficient data on clinical status and/or ADA. This omission did not significantly change the results.

RESUME OF RADIOGRAPHIC DATA ON 49 PATIENTS WITH CID
(Italicized numbers indicate patients with absent red cell ADA.)

		(A) ADA RBC NEG + ADA RBC POS	(B) ADA RBC NEG ONLY
VI.	Pneumonia (continued) 41, *42*, 44, 51, *54*, 56, <u>*57*</u>, 64, 65, 67, 68, 70, *71*, 75, 76, 77, <u>*78*</u>, *84*		
VII.	Thickening of walls of major bronchi	29	
VIII.	Moderate to marked prominence of small bronchi and bronchioli W.S. *1, 2, 3, 4, 37, 53, 54*, 75, 76, 77, <u>*78*</u>, *80, 81*	13	9
IX.	Probable air trapping W.S. *2*, 46, 64, *71*	4	2
X.	Atelectasis	5	0
XI.	Pleural effusion W.S. 69	1	

GASTROINTESTINAL TRACT

XII.	Thickening of valvulae conniventes and/or widening of small bowel W.S. *2*, 69, 70, 75, 76, 77	6	1

BONE

XIII.	Concavity and flaring of anterior rib ends W.S. *3*, <u>*9*</u>, *37, 42, 53, 54*, <u>*57, 78*</u>, *84*	9	9

276

RESUME OF RADIOGRAPHIC DATA ON 49 PATIENTS WITH CID
(Italicized numbers indicate patients with absent red cell ADA.)

		(A) ADA RBC NEG + ADA RBC POS	(B) ADA RBC NEG ONLY
XIV.	Abnormal bony pelvis W.S. *3, 37, 42, 53, 54*	5	5
XV.	Abnormal contour of and articulation of posterior ribs and transverse processes W.S. *37, 42, 53, 54, 57*	5	5
XVI.	Platyspondyly (flat vertebral bodies) W.S. *37, 42, 53, 54*	4	4
XVII.	Thick growth arrest strata W.S. *37, 53, 82*	3	3
XVIII.	Hyperradiolucency of bone ends (trabecular poverty) W.S. *3, 42*	2	2
XIX.	Slight kyphos and beaking of lumbar bodies W.S. *37, 53, 70*	3	2
XX.	Osteoporosis W.S. 43, *53,* 66, 75, 76, 77, *78, 82*	8	3
XXI.	Diminished bone age	3	
XXII.	Abnormal number of ribs (A) 13 ribs W.S. *2* (B) 11 ribs W.S. 68	2 1 1	1 1 0
XXIII.	Fractures of vertebral bodies W.S. 66	1	0

277

PATHOLOGICAL FINDINGS

Jan Huber
John Kersey

Adequate tissue and ADA data were available on nine of the forty autopsied cases we reviewed. In the thymus we looked for dysplasia (an undifferentiated appearance of thymus epithelium) which must be distinguished from extreme involution. This central medullary epithelium consists of large eosinophilic cells with large oval nuclei which form the Hassall bodies after its presumed function has been performed. The thymus can become depleted under a number of circumstances; it is not a specific sign of immune deficiency. Thus, lymphocytes can disappear quickly, causing the thymus to decrease in size following radiation, cortisone, cystostatic drug treatment and severe stress. In order to distinguish the thymus response to drugs and stress from the thymus in immune deficiency disorders, we looked at the difference between the cortex and the medulla, particularly the medullary epithelium.

In the spleen we looked for periarteriolar lymphocyte sheaths, cuffs of lymphocytes around the arteriole, for the presence of follicles and follicle centers and plasma cells.

In the lymph nodes we looked at the general architecture and specifically for follicles and centers (B cell area), pericortical and deep cortex (T cell area) and for plasma cells along the medullary sinuses.

We examined the Peyer's patches and tonsils. Sometimes one does not find organized Peyer's patches but small accumulations of lymphocytes scattered throughout the mucosa. We looked for plasma cells in the mucosa, particularly for signs of graft versus host (GVH) reaction which sometimes destroys the deeper parts of the crypts.

In the lungs we checked for the presence of virus, fungi, bacteria, pneumocystis carinii and for signs of malignancy.

We examined the skin particularly for the presence of GVH reaction; the bone marrow; the liver, also for GVH reaction in the portal triads; kidneys and salivary glands for cytomegalovirus and other organisms. We were, of course, aware of the possibility of malignancy, particularly of the lymphoreticular system.

There were no significant differences in the lymph nodes or skin from patients with or without ADA activity.

We were particularly concerned with the cells of the lymphoid series although, of course, other cell lines also can be affected. The heavy cell traffic from the bone marrow to the various lymphatic organs is reflected in organ morphology.

In the normal thymus of an infant, the cortex is filled with lymphocytes and the medulla with specialized epithelium and Hassall bodies. There is little connective tissue between the lobules (Fig. 1). In the thymus of a 22 week old fetus, the findings are the same with the lobules connected by a stalk area. Hassall bodies are already present (Fig. 2). In the thymus from a child who had been ill for 30 hours, the thymus has undergone lymphoid depletion without the lobular shrinkage characteristic of involution (Fig. 3). The cortex is mottled, presenting a starry-sky appearance. The lymphocytes are engulfed by macrophages and within a couple of days the whole cortex may become devoid of lymphoid cells (Fig. 4). Thus, the presence or absence of lymphoid cells in the thymus is not a good criterion for immune deficiency; lymphoid depletion may occur in children under any kind of stress. Five days after the onset of stress we see the empty cortex and medulla, many Hassall bodies, shrinkage of the lobules and only a few lymphoid cells (Fig. 5). Blood vessels remain present and are relatively large. In the medulla there is a large amount of epithelium and many Hassall bodies (Fig. 6). In our opinion, the latter are garbage bags and their presence indicates past activity of the central medullary epithelium. Sometimes one sees a bizarre picture of the central epithelium with extremely large and cystic Hassall bodies (Fig. 7). The thymus from a child with leukemia treated with large doses of cortisone showed extreme thymic involution such as might be found in a much older person of 60 or 70 years (Fig. 8).

There are two types of epithelium in the thymus (Fig. 9). There is the central epithelium with large eosinophilic cells which form the Hassall bodies and there is the line of undifferentiated epithelium along the periphery of the lobules. This is easy to see in the half depleted thymus. After the central epithelium has performed its function, the cells undergo atrophy, hyalinization, keratinization and eventually form a Hassall body. The center undergoes lysis and the contents are removed. Hassall bodies are constantly being formed and eliminated, especially under antigenic stimulation.

In children with combined immune deficiency disease, the thymus can always be found if searched for carefully. The organ is usually small, weighing one or two grams and if you account for the fat, connective tissue and vessels, the parenchyma may only weigh one half a gram. In children with CID and *normal* erythrocyte ADA activity, no differentiation between cortex and

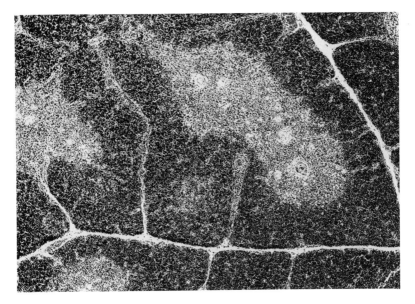

Figure 1

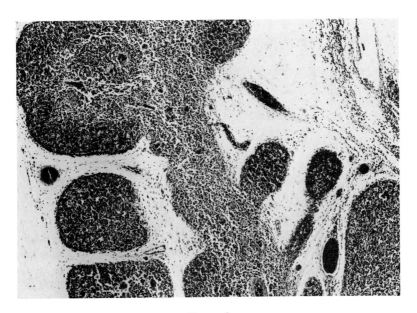

Figure 2

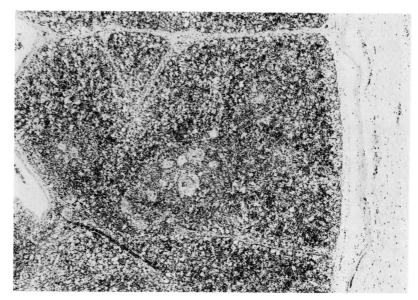

Figure 3

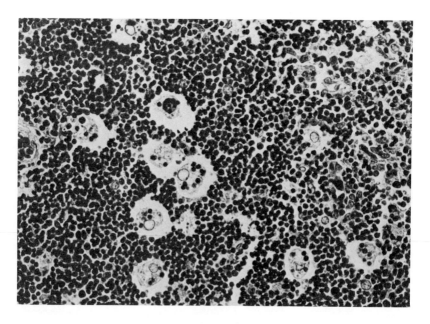

Figure 4

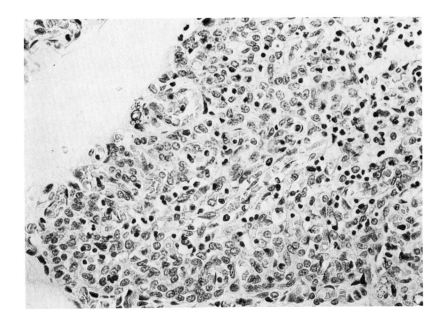

Figure 5

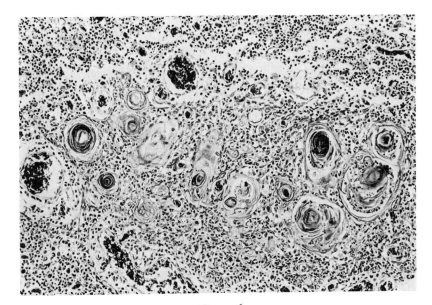

Figure 6

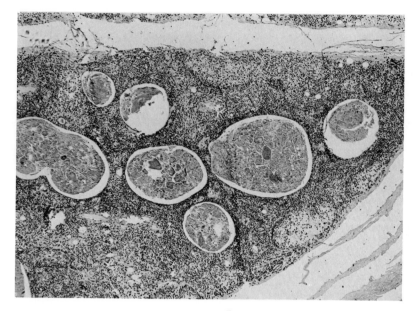

Figure 7

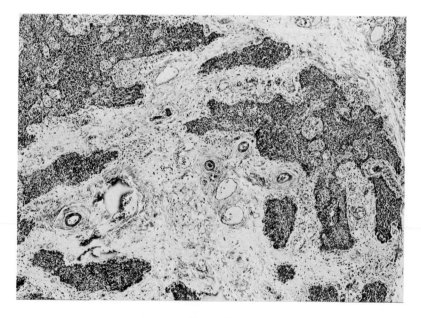

Figure 8

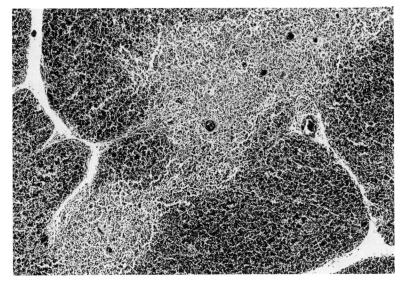

Figure 9

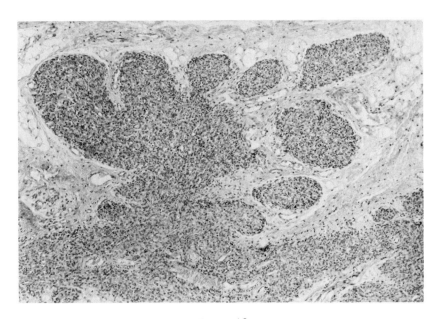

Figure 10

medulla was found and Hassall bodies were absent. Only a few lymphocytes were present (Fig. 10 and 11). The primitive embryonal-looking undifferentiated epithelium formed little rosettes, each surrounded by a PAS positive basement membrane and lacked medullary epithelium (Fig. 12). This is the picture described previously in so-called classical CID.

In patients with CID and *absence* of ADA activity in the red blood cells (Workshop Nos. 1, 2, 3, 57 and 71), we did not see the embryonal type of thymus, as described above, but rather a picture of extreme thymic involution. Thymus atrophy was particularly marked in the differentiated central epithelium. Nevertheless, Hassall corpuscles could be found. The undifferentiated epithelium extended for long stretches but one could observe small areas in this gland that had a different appearance (Fig. 13 and 14). The cells and nuclei were larger and may represent some sort of differentiation of the epithelium. The large cells develop into Hassall bodies after having served their function. Numerous large blood vessels were seen in the thymic interstitium. Thus, the thymuses in the cases without ADA red cell activity had the appearance of a normal but involuted thymus.

On a histological basis, we could not distinguish the spleen, lymph nodes, gastrointestinal tract, bone marrow and other organs of patients with ADA activity from those without ADA activity.

Most of the material submitted to us was obtained post-mortem. In the future, we should be able to obtain more information from lymph nodes taken ante-mortem, using more sophisticated diagnostic methods. We should apply enzyme histochemistry and modifications of rosetting techniques in order to distinguish between B and T cell areas. Eventually, we would like to be able to tell if a gland from a patient, properly stimulated by a known antigen and at a standard time after stimulation, will, for instance, show so much of its volume being taken by the B cell areas and so much in the T cell areas. We will have to establish a range of normal variation in order to be able to give a sound idea of what constitutes a deficient lymph node. Also, immunofluorescence may give us an idea of the capabilities of the cells to produce immunoglobulins. Thymus biopsies may be valuable although they will, of course, only represent a part of the thymus gland and thus introduce a sampling error.

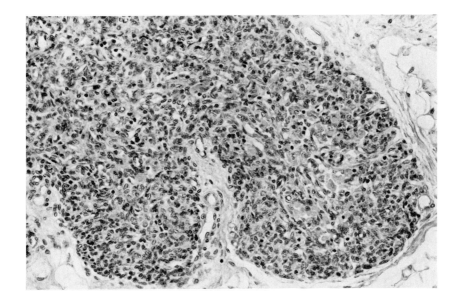

Figure 11

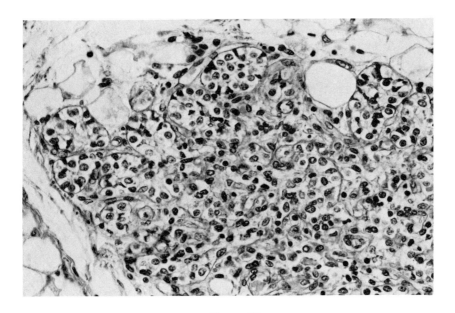

Figure 12

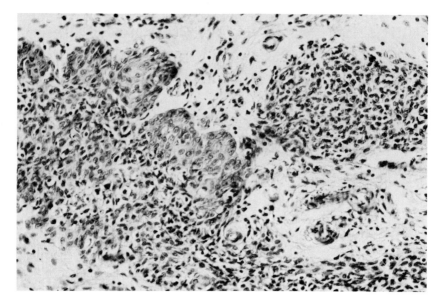

Figure 13

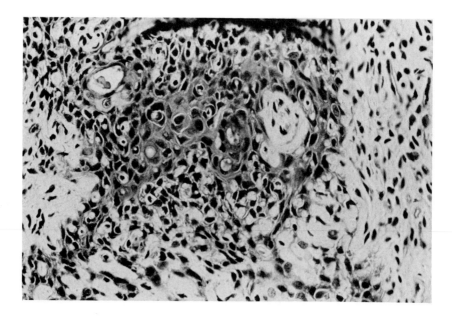

Figure 14

METHODS FOR ASSAY OF ADENOSINE DEAMINASE ACTIVITY

Bernard Pollara

A number of relatively simple and useful methods are available for the assay of adenosine deaminase activity in biological materials. The methods are specific and relatively sensitive.

The diagnosis of ADA deficiency as described by Dr. Giblett[1] was first made using erythrocyte lysates and a starch gel electrophoresis technique.[2] In our studies we attempted to obtain erythrocytes; if these were unavailable, we used stored serum for ADA determinations. Since many of the patients had died, only stored serum samples were available and these were analyzed using Goldberg's method.[3] The results of our studies on serum proved to be fairly reproducible, though other laboratories have found this assay unreliable. Variables such as enzyme instability, variation in storage temperature of serum, possible bacterial contamination, etc., made the precise retrospective diagnosis of ADA deficiency on serum unacceptable to Workshop participants and it was therefore agreed that only those patients in whom erythrocyte ADA was absent would be considered in the ADA deficient group.

The diagnosis of ADA deficiency may be positively and reliably made by analysis of erythrocyte ADA activity by any of the methods discussed below.

Aside from the starch gel technique, two main methods were employed: one in which conversion of adenosine (added to substrate) to inosine results in a spectral shift and resultant decline in absorbancy at 265 nanometers.[4] This method is reliable and reproducible but requires a good ultraviolet spectrophotometer, preferably with a continuous recording device.

The other is a more sensitive spectral assay which I and others prefer.[5] The adenosine to inosine reaction is coupled by adding exogenous xanthine oxidase, yielding uric acid as the final product with a consequent rise in absorbancy at 293 nanometers. In this instance, product information is measured rather than substrate disappearance. Erythrocytes contain adequate nucleoside phosphorylase so that this step is not rate limiting; in lymphocytes, however, nucleoside phosphorylase may be rate limiting. It is difficult to obtain pure nucleoside phosphorylase, so that the preferred assay for lymphocyte ADA is the Kalckar method.[4]

For those laboratories where ultraviolet range spectrophotometers are not available, a specific ammonia release method[6] may be employed. Other variations or modifications have been used, changing incubation times or amounts of substrate, but the results, at least for erythrocytes, have been consistent.

If strict quantitative data is to be obtained, all laboratories should measure ADA activity on a control population. A uniform method of expressing ADA activity should be adapted to facilitate comparisons of results between laboratories. We have expressed our results (for erythrocyte lysates) in terms of micromoles of substrate turned over per minute per unit of absorbance at 540 nanometers. Enzyme activity is usually expressed in terms of moles or micromoles of substrate turned per minute per milligram of protein. If one could rely on hemoglobin determinations, the result could be expressed in relation to grams % hemoglobin. This would be preferable but the variation in analyzing for hemoglobin concentrate is a possible source of considerable error.

A more sensitive and highly specific ^{14}C adenosine technique was employed to analyze tissue ADA activity in one of the deceased patients. We have been using a modification of this method. The products are separated by thin layer chromatography and identified by developing a radioautogram. This is an exquisitely sensitive method which confirmed the spectral analyses on the Albany patient and should prove valuable to resolve questions of residual tissue or fibroblast activity.

Attempts to detect the heterozygote state by quantitation of the enzyme level was not uniformly successful. In studies of the families of the Halifax and Birmingham patients, the presumed carrier parents did not all segregate with low ADA activity. All were greater than one standard deviation but none greater than two standard deviations below the mean. In fact, three mothers of the ADA deficient patients considered by the Workshop had erythrocyte ADA levels that were within the normal range.

To summarize, the main method of diagnosing ADA deficiency is by analyses of ADA activity in erythrocytes. A number of simple and rapid methods are available. These techniques can also be used to determine ADA activity in other cells and tissues.

REFERENCES

1. E.R. Giblett, This Symposium, p.

2. N. Spencer, D.A. Hopkinson and H. Harris, *Ann. Hum. Genet. 32,* 9, 1968.

3. D.M. Goldberg, *Br. Med. Bull. 1,* 353, 1965.

4. H.M. Kalckar, *J. Biol. Chem. 167,* 461, 1947.

5. D.A. Hopkinson, P.J.L. Cook and H. Harris, *Ann. Hum. Genet. 32,* 362, 1969.

6. H. Harker, *Scand. J. Clin. Lab. Invest. 16,* 570, 1964.

7. M.B. van der Weyden, R.H. Buckley and W.N. Kelley, *Biochem. Biophys. Res. Comm. 57,* 590, 1974.

SUMMARY OF THERAPY IN ADA DEFICIENT PATIENTS

Richard Hong

Only patients with RBC ADA deficiency were considered. The "normal" Kalahari Bushman[1] was not included. The patients were arbitrarily divided into two groups, those in whom the diagnosis of combined immunodeficiency disease (CID) was established as set forth in another section of the Workshop and another group, variable immunodeficiency (VID), in which the immunoglobulin and/or T cell deficiencies seem less profound. Table 1 shows the results of liver, thymus and bone marrow transplants upon the clinical status and upon the erythrocyte ADA levels in CID patients. The most striking result in this series is the report of the partial restoration of both B and T cell function in the Birmingham patient as reported earlier in detail by Dr. Keightley.* Further comment on this case will be made later.

Table 2 summarizes the results in the patients with variable immunodeficiency and comprises four patients. Table 3 represents the overall summary of treatment in all groups. Of interest here is that, with the exception of the Birmingham case, liver transplant and thymus transplant were uniformly unsuccessful. Marrow takes were successful in a total of 2 out of 5 instances with partial response in two more. Of interest in this regard is the successful marrow transplant in one of Rosen's cases (WS. No. 80) in which the donor was an ADA deficient heterozygote and there has been no change in ADA status of the recipient. However, that patient is clinically cured; thus, as in ADA normals, successful marrow take results in a normal functioning child. It is also of interest to note at this point that one patient transplanted by Rosen (WS. No. 81) did not have a take, which may be attributed to a small amount of host T cell activity as indicated by the very low PHA response. Nevertheless, this individual's

---

*R. Keightley, this Symposium, p.

293

TABLE 1

Results of Transplant; CID Patients with ADA Deficiency

Workshop Number	Liver B.[b]	Liver T.[b]	Thymus	Bone Marrow B.	Bone Marrow T.	ADA[a]	Status
1					P[c]	—	D[e]
3			No treatment				
37	P	P (9 wk)[d]				+	L[e]
42			No treatment				D
53	No[c]	No (12–15 wk)				—	L
54			No treatment				L
82				Yes[c]	Yes	—	L

a ADA, erythrocyte adenosine deaminase levels after transplant
b B, B cell take; T, T cell take
c P = partial take; Yes = complete take; No = no take
d Age of fetal tissue
e D = dead; L = living

294

TABLE 2

Results of Transplant; VID Patients with ADA Deficiency

Workshop Number	Liver B.	T.	Thymus	Bone Marrow B.	T.	T.F.[a]	ADA	Status
2	No(2)[b]	No(2)	No(4)	Yes	No	No x 10	+ (s)	D
71			P		Yes		−	D
80				Yes	Yes		−	L
81				No	No		−	L

Symbols as in Table 1; also

a TF = transfer factor

b Numbers of trials attempted

cellular immunity tests have improved slowly with time and the patient is still alive at the age of 13 months.

The success with the liver is especially unique in the whole history of reconstitution efforts in combined immunodeficiency diseases.[2] Reasons for this surprising result may be that the fetal donor was quite young — nine weeks. It is possible that there is a very short period during intrauterine life when the fetal liver contains sufficient amounts of stem cells to provide appropriate reconstitution and that employment of liver at periods after this time results in failure. The ability of the transplant to be accomplished rapidly after obtaining the specimen may also have played a significant role. Tissues which have been shipped long distances may have suffered too much cell damage to be able to effect a reconstitution. Finally, there is a distinct possibility that the basic disorder (i.e., ADA deficiency) permitted the success and that, in fact, a transplant not of lymphopoietic stem cells but of some usable source of adenosine deaminase or another appropriate chemical agent may have been operative in this situation. Failure of the lymphocytes in the patient to demonstrate measurable ADA at this time speaks against that hypothesis, however.

On the basis of the results as shown in the tables and from results of transplants which have been employed in the past, one might arrive at a proposal for therapeutic strategy in patients with combined immunodeficiency (Table 4). I think all would agree that matched bone marrow is still the treatment of choice and has met with the most unequivocal and long-lasting results. Recent exciting experiences reported from Denmark[3] indicate that one should now look even outside of the siblings for the possibility of matched donors and this increases the number of possibilities of reconstitution appreciably. Secondly, the use of fetal liver must be completely re-examined utilizing fetuses of this younger age group with the early installation of the product. As a third modality, we are impressed that the experiences of Ammann[4] and ourselves[5] indicate that in non-DiGeorge patients the best results of thymic transplantation have been associated with the previous administration of transfer factor. It is entirely possible that in some as yet undefined way transfer factor has some adjunctive or helpful function in preparing either the thymus or the patient to derive greater benefit from the transplant.

In the particular situation of ADA deficiency, one is intrigued by the possibility of an enzymatic reconstitution. The experience in Fabry's disease where a transplanted kidney was able to effect a reconstitution is extremely provocative in this regard.[6] The ability to isolate enzymes in a pure form is certainly within the realm of technical capability today and, again, in Fabry's disease reconstitution by this direct approach has been possible.[7] Finally, one

TABLE 3

Summary of Transplants — All Patients

	Liver	Thymus	Marrow	ADA Conversion	Alive
CID (6)[a]	1/2[b]	—	1+/2[c]	1	4
VID (4)	0/1	0/2	1+/3	1	4

a Number of patients
b Number of takes/number of attempts
c 1+ = 1 complete take, some partial takes

TABLE 4

Therapeutic Strategy

1. Matched bone marrow (even non-sib)

2. Fetal liver

3. Transfer factor and thymus

4. Enzymatic reconstitution — kidney? wbc?

5. Chemical manipulation

can predict that the kind of chemical manipulation that has been seen in many enzyme deficiencies, such as hereditary orotic aciduria in which the megalo-blastic anemia is very nicely corrected by the administration of uridine, will be accomplished in ADA deficiency.[8]

In closing, I would like to offer a unitary hypothesis which may serve to bring together the wealth of information which has been provided at this Workshop and Symposium by the geneticists, the biochemists and the immunologists. There have been two major observations reported here which seem to single out the ADA deficient patients. The first is a clear demonstration in the Detroit case that thymic tissue was present and demonstrated radiographically during the first year of life in their patient. Secondly, Dr. Huber has, without prior knowledge of the status of the enzyme levels, found a common morphologic appearance to the thymuses of the patients with ADA deficiency. The finding described indicated that the thymus, as Dr. Huber says, "had seen better days". It thus appears that the thymic tissue of the patients with ADA deficiency may have undergone some process which slowly caused its decrease in size and ostensible function. There is precedent for gradual loss of thymic function and thymic tissue. In the experimental situation which was studied by Ekstedt,[9] the injection of sterile vaccines into the thymus of normal mice within the first six hours after birth resulted in severe lymphoid depletion and thymic atrophy with a resultant severe wasting disease of the animals. It was important in this model that the injection be made very early after birth, which means that an assault upon normal lymphoid tissues must begin early in life. In the human situation, it has been shown in diseases such as ataxia telangiectasia and Wiskott-Aldrich that there is a decrease in lymphoid capability and alteration in morphology with time.[10] Another example occurred in two siblings with onset in the second year of life.[10] This phenomenon of gradual wastage of the lymphoid apparatus has been termed "immunologic attrition". I think from the evidence which has been presented at this Symposium one could surmise that the accumulation of toxic products as a result of the ADA deficiency could well result in the prevention of appropriate lymphoid proliferation and the inability to preserve the original clonal mass with which the child was endowed. It is quite unlikely that this accumulation may have begun *in utero*. The end result of this constant attack upon the lymphoid tissue is to render it incapable of responding appropriately to the antigenic stimulation which is a necessary part of post-natal life. As a result, the lymphoid tissue becomes progressively more depleted. The immunologic function wanes and at death there is a tremendous paucity of lymphoid tissue. However, there persists a remnant of the original thymic central epithelium, indicating that the defect

298

was not intrinsic in the thymic epithelium but, in fact, was a result of a continuous assault on lymphocyte precursors. The nature of the toxic product is as yet unknown. It seems not to be adenosine nor any of the related nucleotides. A suggestion has been made that perhaps it is PRPP.

The high degree of associated bony defects may represent another tissue unable to proliferate appropriately in this milieu.

Whatever the reason, whatever the mechanism, the opening of the study of immunologic deficiency to the precise tools of the biochemist begins a most exciting chapter in the field of immunologic deficiency diseases.

REFERENCES

1. T. Jenkins, *Lancet II,* 736, 1973.

2. R.H. Buckley, *in* Progress in Immunology, B. Amos (Ed.), p. 1061, Academic Press, New York, 1973.

3. Copenhagen Study Group of Immunodeficiencies, *Lancet I,* 1146, 1973.

4. A.J. Ammann, D.W. Wara, S. Salmon and H. Perkins, *New Eng. J. Med. 289,* 5, 1973.

5. R. Hong, *in* Proceedings of the Second International Workshop on Primary Immunodeficiency Diseases in Man, St. Petersburg, Florida, 1973.

6. R.J. Desnick, K.Y. Allen, R.L. Simmons, J.S. Najarian and W. Krivit, *J. Lab. Clin. Med. 78,* 989, 1971.

7. R.O. Brady, J.F. Tallman, W.G. Johnson, A.E. Gal, W.R. Leahy, J.M. Quirk and A.S. Dekaban, *New Eng. J. Med. 289,* 9, 1973.

8. L.H. Smith, C.M. Huguley, Jr. and J.A. Bain, *in* The Metabolic Basis of Inherited Disease, J.B. Stanbury, J.B. Wyngaarden and D.S. Fredrickson (Eds.), p. 1003, McGraw-Hill Book Company, New York, 1972.

9. R.D. Ekstedt and L.L. Hayes, *J. Immun. 98,* 110, 1967.

10. A.J. Ammann and R. Hong, *in* Immunologic Disorders in Infants and Children, E.R. Stiehm and V. Fulginiti (Eds.), p. 236, W.B. Saunders Co., Philadelphia, 1973.

DISCUSSION

DR. ALBERTINI: The evidence seems to indicate that this is a disease determined by a single gene and is autosomal. However, since the South African patient raises the question of somatic cell mosaicism, I wonder if the fibroblasts from mothers of ADA deficient boys have been looked at for mosaicism which you could potentially expect if there were a sex-linked form of this, analogous to the mosaicism of Lesch-Nyhan mothers.

DR. WOLFSON: I wanted to comment on Dr. Hong's beautiful presentation and say that he is quite right. Dr. Cross and I excluded other abnormalities so as not to confuse things. Experience will tell us whether what we have presented really presents a clear and homogenous aspect of a syndrome or whether there will be descriptions of additional findings and variations.

You may have heard what one witty individual said when asked if he had discovered something new: "What, after all, can be new," he said, "to a generation that has seen the polar ice from below, the moon from above and Marilyn Monroe from the side." My final comment is that much new has indeed occurred here.

DR. MEUWISSEN: Are there any clinical syndromes that radiologically resemble what you have described?

DR. WOLFSON: Probably the one syndrome that this resembles the most, and then only superficially, is achondroplasia. There are others. The association of abnormalities as has occurred in our patients appears to be distinctive.

I did call Dr. Leonard Langer on the telephone and described what we have seen. He is a highly regarded authority on the radiographic findings in dwarfism and it was his view that this constellation of findings is distinctive.

DR. PICKERING: Someone has asked for comments on the possibility of using red cells that are high in ADA content or plasma that is high in ADA content in the treatment of this syndrome. We have given ADA positive whole blood to our patient on at least three occasions and we haven't seen changes in any immunological parameters.

GEORGE L. TRITSCH (Roswell Park Memorial Institute, Buffalo, New York): I would like to comment on the finding of lack of adenosine deaminase activity. The assays used all implied a high substrate concentration. In some of the tissues, inosine deaminase is inhibited by adenosine levels and possibly this lack of ADA activity could simply be due to inhibitors present in the reaction mixtures. Some of the most potent inhibitors of enzymes are the modified nucleosides which occur via DNA and RNA turnover in the cells and some of these materials are very potent or competitive inhibitors of enzymes.

DR. POLLARA: I think the things you mentioned have been considered at one time or another by each of us singly and some of us collectively. The assay conditions employed in the spectrophotometric methods are such that we are working at optimum concentrations. Furthermore, experiments in which we've mixed lysates, lymphocytes and red cells from the affected patient with those of normal individuals, have never inhibited those reactions.

DR. PARKS: I would like to propose a relatively simple screening procedure that I believe would be more specific than the method presented at this meeting, which uses the pH change caused by ammonia liberated during ADA reaction. This would be based on the fact that in human erythrocytes the activity of purine nucleoside phosphorylase (PNPase) is about 100 times greater than that of adenosine deaminase. For example, we find that ADA activity normally is in the range of 0.15 to 0.25 μM units per ml of RBC's. Therefore, if hemolysates are added to a solution containing adenosine, orthophosphate, xanthine oxidase and an electron-accepting dye such as dichlorophenol indophenol a color change should occur and the rate of change would be dependent on the concentration of adenosine deaminase. The reaction sequence would be: adenosine to inosine by the ADA reaction; inosine reacting with PNPase to form hypoxanthine; hypoxanthine reacting with xanthine oxidase to form uric acid, coupled with the transfer of electrons to the indicator dye. My guess is that a practical test could be developed for small quantities of blood. Of course, it would be necessary to select a redox dye for which the color change could be easily detected against the background color of hemoglobin.

DR. MOORE: One advantage of the method I presented is that you can use the filter paper spots instead of a liquid form and is much easier to collect.

DR. PARKS: I don't know whether the test, as I have suggested it, could be performed by a filter paper method because I don't know whether PNPase in the red cells would survive drying on filter paper. Of course, that would have to be tested. However, PNPase is very easy to isolate in quite large quantities from erythrocytes and the complete separation of adenosine deaminase from PNPase is also simple. We have reported a large-scale preparation procedure for the isolation of a number of enzymes, including PNPase, from outdated blood-bank red cells and the Enzyme Center at Tufts University Medical School has carried out this method for us several times (K.C. Agarwal, E.M. Scholar, R.P. Agarwal and R.E. Parks, Jr., *Biochem. Pharmacol. 20,* 1341, 1971). You can also purchase crystalline beef spleen purine nucleoside phosphorylase and xanthine oxidase from bovine milk is inexpensive. Therefore, there should be little problem in adding filter paper spots to a solution containing both of these enzymes plus the appropriate substrates, indicator dyes, etc. If sufficient adenosine deaminase has survived to permit detection via the pH change method, there also should be enough to permit detection by the method that I suggest. Also, since all of the necessary agents may be obtained at relatively modest cost, the expense of the method should not be a problem.

OVERVIEW

Kurt Hirschhorn

I am reminded at this state of the ADA story of events in the late 1950's, when a group of immunologists, serologists, biochemists and geneticists got together and pooled their observations and calculations to solve a basic problem in biology; namely, the nature of the ABO blood groups. If one reads the history of that synthesis, one can see that the information from each of these groups would never have been sufficient to resolve the question of what the ABO blood groups are. I think we are seeing this here – a mingling of disciplines to resolve a problem.

I would like to give you briefly my biased impressions of the various talks and stress one or two points in each of the presentations, with occasional side comments.

Dr. Porter introduced the word that became a major theme of the Symposium, the word *heterogeneity* and, later on, Dr. Pollara and others made it clear that heterogeneity has two ends to its spectrum – genetic and environmental – and these may be rather difficult to separate. There may be some methods that will help us to do this. Dr. Porter also made it clear that inborn errors are really an end of a spectrum of polymorphism – of human variation. They happen to be those that we can detect on the basis of disease in our present environment. Nevertheless, we must remember that each of us is quite different from the other and that this reflects on the question that was asked: "What is normal?".

The discovery of inborn errors of metabolism as specific enzyme defects is, by now, a weekly event that Dr. Porter showed in an exponentially rising curve. Therefore, to the geneticist, the finding of ADA deficiency is just another inborn error and I think it is the combination of talents that has made this finding biologically meaningful.

Dr. Litwin gave us a fine review of the genetics of the immune response, divided into the antibody response and the cellular immune response. I wish that he had included a theme that recurred several times during the Symposium – the mixed lymphocyte culture response. Whether this is, in fact, part and parcel of the immune response complex or a separate locus that happens to be closely linked, I think it is going to be pertinent. We later heard from Dr. Cohen that there may be a dissociation between mixed lymphocyte culture response and lymphocyte mediated cytotoxicity to complicate that which Dr. Litwin calls the immune response histocompatibility genetic region. The mixed lymphocyte culture which I have heard proposed several times as the real test of histocompatibility for selection of bone marrow donors and probably for donors of other organs was predicted in 1963[1] when we described this test and compared it to the cross-match in blood transfusion. HLA, just like ABO typing, may be similar to dissociation in some of the minor blood groups; if one needs to give a transfusion, one doesn't pay much attention to these and, in fact, most of the time one doesn't even type for them. But the cross-match will tell you whether there is an incompatibility with some of these other blood groups that may not have been detected in actual typing and which may be important for the "take" of the transfusion and, in corollary, the "take" of the organ.

Another aspect that should be stressed is the role of various genetic factors in maturation and differentiation of the cells. We really know nothing of the genetic control of differentiation of any organ. This probably remains the most talked about problem in human and general biology. I think this is perhaps where some of the inherited immune deficiency diseases may give us clues.

One other aspect that perhaps was not sufficiently stressed is that portion of the immune response that depends upon T and B cell interaction. Once again, this may turn out to be a central problem in combined immunodeficiency and perhaps even in some of the other immunodeficiency states. For example, the fact that cells from certain patients with agammablobulinemia can make immunoglobulin *in vitro* but not *in vivo*, makes one think that perhaps the defect is in the T − B cell interaction, as Dr. Litwin implied, rather than primarily in the B cell.

Dr. Rosen's excellent review of the immunodeficiency diseases leads me to speculate that X-linked thymic alymphoplasia, X-linked thrombocytopenia and Wiskott-Aldrich syndrome might represent alleles at one X-linked locus that has something to do with bone marrow maturation. Different mutations at this locus may interfere at different steps during the maturation of bone marrow cells. I think it would be worthwhile to study patients with each of these conditions for what their bone marrow cells can do to *in vitro* differentiation of other bone marrow cells that may have defects earlier on. Can they push them on to a certain step of maturation? Can we isolate some factor from bone marrow that is, in fact, a differentiating factor which is determined by the gene in the X-chromosome?

I must draw attention to the importance of environmental influences. We are all aware that no gene operates without the appropriate environment. If we had a taboo against eating dairy products and drinking milk, we would never know about galactosemia. We must always keep this in mind. Modification by environment is important, not only in terms of what we usually consider as the environment but, as Dr. Pollara mentioned, the maternal-fetal unit environment and perhaps even the intrafetal environment as determined by the general genetic makeup of the fetus as a background against which mutation is acting.

Dr. Fox's talk on purine metabolism was most valuable and I will treasure his diagram with the notes that I made during his talk, in order to attempt to understand all the various cycles that operate in this system.

I think Dr. Nyhan's presentation of the Lesch-Nyhan syndrome can teach us many lessons. The major one, to me as a geneticist, is that in collecting data about various diseases and about various normal metabolic steps, one is impressed by how much we learn about normal physiology and normal biochemistry as a result of inborn errors of metabolism. I only need remind you that the amino acid cystine — the first amino acid discovered — was found in a cystine stone from a patient with cystinuria. In fact, normal thyroid metabolism was only elucidated on the basis of the various inborn errors of thyroid metabolism. I think we are now beginning to see this in nucleotide metabolism as taught us initially by the Lesch-Nyhan syndrome and, hopefully, now with some of the elegant studies described from ADA deficiency.

Dr. Meuwissen's description of the first case is of great value. His questions as to whether CID causes ADA deficiency, ADA deficiency causes CID, the two are independent or, as Dr. Nyhan added, a common factor causes both is, of course, proper scientific method in trying to resolve the problem. I think he satisfied us that CID most likely cannot cause adenosine deaminase deficiency. I think we have to eliminate the question of independent causation completely because in the thousands of individual studies at the Galton laboratory by Hopkinson, Harris and their collaborators, deficient individuals have not been found, which means that the deficiency *per se* is rare. To ask now for two rare events, combined immunodeficiency disease and ADA deficiency, to occur together in the number of cases we have now seen, is asking too much of coincidence.

As to a common factor causing both CID and ADA deficiency, the only one I can conceive of is the one that Dr. Giblett has already hopefully put to rest; that is, deletion. I understand that Dr. Gerald has now done rather careful chromosome banding studies to search for a major deletion in the heterozygotes for ADA deficiency and, in the cases that Drs. Meuwissen and Pollara kindly obtained for us, we find that the two number 20 chromosomes (assuming, as we have heard from Dr. Gerald and others, that ADA is on number 20) are completely alike. In fact, we have also looked at all the karyotypes and have not found any differences with quite careful and successful banding studies. This doesn't eliminate a small deletion by any means, but, at least, it is not a sizable one. We have heard from Dr. Cohen and the description of her family that the heterozygotes for ADA deficiency, at least in her family, have a full house of HLA antigens. In other words, they have four antigens and what one would expect if this were due to a deletion of the region containing HLA is that they would only have 2 antigens, representing one chromosome in that region and not two. This is another piece of evidence against deletion.

Dr. Gerald introduced us to the most powerful tool for gene mapping; that is, cell hybridization. From this information, I think the entire commentary regarding HLA and deletion becomes superfluous because he says HLA is on chromosome 6 and ADA is on 20. Perhaps we should retain a bit of caution on this point. Dr. Gerald expressed this himself and pointed out that chromosome 20 is a small one and, therefore, retained more frequently in the hybrids. We also have to remember that the placement of HLA is dependent upon a single study which places the locus 3 for phosphoglucomutase (PGM3) on 6 and because of the reasonable linkage information from family data between HLA and PGM3, we have now placed HLA on 6. This is not fully confirmed at this time.

Dr. Giblett gave us an excellent review of the genetics of ADA and I completely agree that the autosomal recessive mode of inheritance of ADA is, by far, the most likely explanation.

We come again to the question of heterogeneity, this time purely from the genetic point of view. I think that the Jenkins case, and conceivably the Cohen cases, demonstrate what we expect to find. The Jenkins case has a deficiency of the enzyme at least in one tissue and is reasonably normal, although I am not completely satisfied that we have all the information that we are going to get on that 12 year old child. The Cohen case appears to be intermediate in severity, at least in the four year old child, and the question of whether some tissue isozymes remain in that child is still open. Such remaining enzyme activity may represent a tissue isozyme, low in activity and altered in its properties. Part of this alteration may be a lack of release from a conversion factor and such a severe alteration so as to change its electrophoretic behavior. I would not be at all surprised to find cases of relative ADA deficiency, homozygous in nature, who do have remaining enzyme activity. We have many such examples of genetic heterogeneity in a whole variety of inborn errors of metabolism and the Lesch-Nyhan syndrome is a perfect example of this where we have within the syndrome a whole variety of mutations resulting in the presence of cross-reacting material with minor activity, others with no activity and if we move one step up to gout patients with HGPRT deficiency, the spectrum is even wider and each family breeds true. This true genetic heterogeneity may account for family to family variation in ADA deficiency.

I think, personally, that if we take the 13 cases that we have heard about, of whom two derive from consanguineous matings, that we might find as many as 24 mutations. Once we are able to isolate any cross-reacting material; that is, the inactive adenosine deaminase protein, and can do amino acid analysis, each mutation is going to be quite different except that within the consanguineous family the two genes will be alike. In all the other families, I think that none of the children are likely to be homozygous. They are probably double heterozygotes for deficient alleles. This is now becoming quite clear in a number of different diseases; for example, in homocystinuria where one finds double heterozygotes for two different defects in cystathionine synthetase that produces the disease of homocystinuria.

Dr. Ressler made us aware of some of the induced, artifactual and natural variations that can be obtained and observed in starch gel. I think that most of his data referred primarily to the red cell form of ADA, including his data on the spleen but I am not completely certain of this.

Dr. Rochelle Hirschhorn's presentation has been adequately commented upon by Dr. Giblett and if I add my praise I will be accused of bias. I think the important points to come from her studies are the strong evidence for one locus defining activity of all the isozymes; evidence for various conversion factors in various tissue, proven in tissues from a deficient patient; and the adenosine inhibition data in her lymphocyte activation work from some years ago. I am reminded, regarding enzyme conversion, of some experiments with Beratis and Seepers we reported from our laboratory a few years ago.[2] Another enzyme, placental alkaline phosphatase, shows polymorphism like red cell ADA and the polymorphism is seen in a set of fast moving isozymes in starch gel. There is a set of slow isozymes which show no polymorphism. First, we were able to show that the slow isozyme could be converted into the fast isozyme and regain its polymorphic genotype of the fetus whose placenta we were studying. Secondly, we could show that the slow bands were considerably larger molecules and, in fact, were made up of several bands of varying larger sizes which were much more heat stable than the fast bands. The slow bands were much less enzymatically active, mole for mole. Therefore, we have a parallel between the tissue and red cell ADA and the slow bands and fast bands of placental alkaline phosphatase. We proposed at the time that what this represents is a storage form of the enzyme (slow bands) which can release an enzyme that is much more active at a time when it is needed. What is more, we proposed a new definition of thermal stability because placental alkaline phosphatase is said to be an enormously heat stable enzyme when, in fact, it is not. The fast bands are quite labile and what happens as you expose the extract to warmth is that you get continuous release from the slow, relatively heat stable enzyme (low activity) fraction of a heat labile enzyme (high activity) fraction and this, when measured as stability, looks as if enzyme activity remains at a constant level. In reality, you are depleting it. If you keep it up long enough you'll have no enzyme left, even though for a long time activity may remain quite constant. I think this is something to be considered here and I will get back to this in terms of ADA.

Dr. Pollara's discussion alluded to this, of course, when he talked about the various methods by which an enzyme defect could cause disease. One of the first things he mentioned was that a precursor may be toxic or that there is an irregularity of the metabolic pathways in that pathways which are not normally active are now activated and that products of such alternate pathways may be toxic or that lack of a product may be the important thing. I don't think we have resolved any of these questions in ADA deficiency.

A fourth mechanism that now has been well studied is that one has an enzyme which cannot properly interact with a cofactor. We have this in the various vitamin dependent diseases such as methylmalmonic aciduria, various forms of homocystinuria, etc., and while I know nothing of any conceivable cofactor requirement for ADA, perhaps eventually some will be shown to exist. I think this needs to be kept in mind.

In order to resolve the question of environmental versus genetic variation we need many families for proper genetic analysis, those with affected sibs, in order to dissect these factors. As was said, an animal model would help.

Dr. Green's exciting talk may have opened up an entirely new aspect of this field with a quite different approach to therapy than the ones Dr. Hong described at the and. I think that his suggestion for pyrimidine starvation as the principal cause of the disease certainly should be pursued by those people who have patients. He suggests that different cell types may get rid of adenosine in different ways and that, therefore, not all the cells are affected in the same way by the same enzyme deficiency. In other words, the metabolism of adenosine needs to be studied in various tissues.

The discussion by Dr. Hadden brought us up to date on the properties of T and B cells, the study of which has become so important in evaluating these patients. He also referred to lymphocyte studies with cyclic AMP and cyclic GMP. These compounds are related to adenosine and its metabolism but certainly it is not clear at this time what the interrelationship is between ADA deficiency and the roles of these cyclic nucleotides in normal lymphocyte metabolism. I think this is well worth examining, perhaps with the use of ADA inhibitors.

Dr. Cohen's studies of the dissociation of CML and MLC in her family are fascinating but I am not certain at this point how this related to ADA deficiency. The fact that her two sibs were somewhat different clinically may help us in assessing some of the genetic and environmental factors.

Dr. Keightley's liver transplant, as Dr. Hong has said, is a stimulating experience that obviously needs a great deal of follow-up and study in order to see what, in fact, has happened and whether this is unique for ADA deficiency. One question is whether in this chimera, created by the liver transplant, the patient's own cells recovered their normal function. This has to be looked at by a variety of genetic methods.

Dr. Moore's screening test sounds like it will be useful and, as I understand it, has already been applied in one area and will probably become part of the multiphasic Guthrie type test, where one blood-stained filter paper can now be used for a number of screening tests. I would like it very much if she and others were to apply themselves to developing a cheap and easy carrier test so that we can find out something about gene frequencies, etc., in the normal population.

The Workshop was very well summarized by Dr. Hong. We are grateful to Dr. Pickering for maintaining his management of the Workshop and to Dr. Hong for reviewing the crucial aspects. Here again, we have collaboration not only between the immunologist, the geneticist and the biochemist but between the people who have to deal with the immediate problem, the clinician, the pathologist, the radiologist, all interacting in a way that should be used for all of the immunodeficiency diseases.

Dr. Hong's comments on forms of therapy were well taken. I would, however, remind him that the Fabry's disease correction with kidney transplant deals with a lysosomal enzyme which is secreted and can exist in the cell in new lysosomes. Whether this can be done with ADA should be easily resolvable by taking ADA negative fibroblasts and exposing them to the enzyme in culture to see whether they take it up.

In summary, I would like to stress a few points. First, what is normal? Our definition of normal is plus or minus 2 and in some cases 3 standard deviations from some mean value. Dr. Porter mentioned the enormous degree of polymorphism in man. Obviously, we are all genetically and biochemically different. If we are going to start looking at where we differ in terms of two standard deviations from a mean and if we look at different characteristics, we are all abnormal in some way. We all carry 3 to 8 genes in single dose for inborn errors of metabolism, therefore, we fall into an abnormal range for a variety of enzymes. Therefore, normal has to be defined just for the aspect you are studying. Even that is difficult because we don't know what the individual's genetic background will do to the expression of a particular polymorphism. If we look at enough polymorphisms in populations with certain common diseases, we may come up with constellations of genotypes that turn out to be more susceptible to these, such as hypertension, diabetes, etc. The same is true for the expression of single gene determinants; those who have been doing animal breeding and using the mathematics for polygenic inheritance, long ago found out that a number of characteristics are determined by additive genes, onto which you can superimpose a so-called dominant effect from a single gene. For example, height in normal individuals follows a normal distribution. If someone has a dominant gene for an achondroplasia, he or she is short. Nevertheless, if we look at all the achondro-plastics, we find a normal distribution curve for the height of achondro-plastics. We have to know what makes a particular achondroplastic or a normal relatively small or not so small. Perhaps some of the gene constellations of the polymorphisms can give us some of these answers.

I would like to summarize my own personal view of how ADA deficiency may work. ADA may exist in tissues as a storage enzyme. I would suspect that if this enzyme is isolated and studied biochemically and compared to red cell ADA, that the conditions for its optimal activity will be biologic nonsense. In other words, these storage enzymes *in vivo* are relatively inactive biologically. When the need arises – and there I like the word recycling rather than salvage – reutilizing adenosine, the active form that is the "red cell" form of the enzyme is released and does its job. Perhaps this can only happen efficiently in certain tissues – there are some tissues in which we don't even find any "red cell" form – and these may be the tissues that go bad in ADA deficiency. We have heard about the lymphoid tissue; we've heard that bone may be involved; we've heard some clues about endocrine difficulties. I am suggesting that we should study intestinal mucosa carefully as to cell kinetics, not just morphologically, to see whether there is an abnormality in this rapidly proliferating organ in ADA deficiency. It may be, of course, that this pathway is only necessary for episodically proliferating cells or in Dr. Green's relatively artifactual system of established cell lines. In other tissues, it may not be so necessary; they may have other mechanisms. If it is needed and if there is no recycling because there is no adenosine deaminase, we get what we have all around us when we have no recycling: pollution. What the pollutant is may not be clear but certainly one of the major lessons from this Symposium is that the most likely answer to ADA deficiency is that something is polluting and leads to death of certain cells.

The last comment relates to something everybody here has been saying: now that we have an enzyme defect for one immunologic deficiency disease, obviously we'll have enzyme defects for all immunologic deficiency diseases. I am not so sure of this because, again, I remind you that we know nothing about differentiation genes. Their products may or may not be enzymes. We may have to go back and study new kinds of enzymes or other proteins in fetal tissues, something that you know is becoming more and more difficult, thanks to some unfavorable publicity. However, I would like to propose to the combined disciplines here that perhaps the next immune deficiency to be resolved is ataxia telangiectasia. I would suggest that we take a close look at all of the known and as yet to be discovered repair enzymes for DNA, to look for a defect in ataxia telangiectasia.

Finally, the most important benefit from this Symposium is the one that I mentioned at the beginning. After 15 years, we have again succeeded in coordinating three disciplines — immunology, biochemistry and genetics — to work jointly on a problem. I think that if we can continue to do this, it will be profitable for us all.

I am sure I speak for the whole audience when I echo Dr. Pickering's gratitude to Drs. Porter, Meuwissen and Pollara for their excellent organization and warm hospitality.

REFERENCES

1.   K. Hirschhorn, F. Bach, R.L. Kolodny, I.L. Firschein and N. Hashem, *Science 242,* 1185, 1963.

2. a. N.G. Beratis, W. Seegers and K. Hirschhorn, *Biochem. Genet. 4,* 689, 1970.

   b. N.G. Beratis, W. Seegers and K. Hirschhorn, *Biochem. Genet. 5,* 367, 1971.

   c. N.G. Beratis and K. Hirschhorn, *Biochem. Genet. 6,* 1, 1972.

313

SUBJECT INDEX

A

Acetylcholine, 173, 176
Achondroplasia, 267, 271, 301, 313
Adenine, 48, 49, 141, 150, 188
  eliminated from cell by excretion, 150
  nucleotide pool, 52
  phosphoribosyltransferase (APRT), 49, 67,
    93, 141
  isozymes, 69
Adenosine, 51, 73, 80, 135, 141, 142, 148,
  149, 189
  ^{14}C, 73
  cycle, 148
  deaminase (ADA), 50, 59, 85, 103, 105,
    117-119, 121, 123-127, 129, 131, 135,
    141, 149, 153, 188, 198
    activity, 73, 109, 125
      during lymphocyte stimulation, 191
      in fibroblasts, 109
    as a regulating agent, 148
    associated with disease, 121
    bands, 115
      multiple, 111
    cases, 105
      cities, 105
    conversion, 118

    of "RBC" ADA isozymes, 124
  deficiency, 11, 26, 73, 85, 86, 136, 166,
    168
    discovery of, 105
    immune disease, 109
    Isoprinosine in, 168
    prenatal diagnosis of, 109, 126
  fibroblasts, 125
  genetic control, 80
  genotypes, 106
  in biological materials, 289
  in calf serum, 142
  inhibition, 197
  in malignancy, 80
  in the newborn, 130
  isozymes, 108, 111, 121, 124, 126, 307,
    309
    in fibroblasts and lymphocytes, 108
    patterns of, 115
    red blood cell, 121, 122
    "tissue specific", 127
  kidney, 111
  loci, 79, 80, 99, 108
  lung, 117
  molecular weight, 117, 119
  phenotypes, 105
    2-1 phenotype, 124

A 5
B 6
C 7
D 8
E 9
F 0
G 1
H 2
I 3
J 4